GROW
A NEW
BRAIN

Also by Alberto Villoldo

Grow a New Body Cookbook

Grow a New Body

The Wisdom Wheel

Power Up Your Brain

The Shaman's Dream Oracle

Mystic Shaman Oracle

Soul Journeying

The Illumination Process

The Heart of the Shaman

The Four Insights

All of the above are available at your local bookstore,
or may be ordered by visiting:

Hay House USA: www.hayhouse.com®
Hay House Australia: www.hayhouse.com.au
Hay House UK: www.hayhouse.co.uk
Hay House India: www.hayhouse.co.in

***

HOW SPIRIT AND POWER PLANTS CAN
PROTECT AND UPGRADE YOUR BRAIN

GROW
A NEW

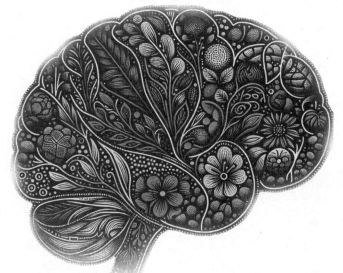

BRAIN

DR. ALBERTO VILLOLDO

HAY HOUSE LLC
Carlsbad, California • New York City
London • Sydney • New Delhi

Published in the United States by: Hay House LLC: www.hayhouse.com˚
Published in Australia by: Hay House Australia Publishing Pty Ltd: www
.hayhouse.com.au • *Published in the United Kingdom by:* Hay House UK Ltd:
www.hayhouse.co.uk • *Published in India by:* Hay House Publishers (India)
Pvt Ltd: www.hayhouse.co.in

Cover design: The Book Designers • *Interior design:* Nick C. Welch

**Cataloging-in-Publication Data is on file
at the Library of Congress**

Hardcover ISBN: 978-1-4019-7318-6
E-book ISBN: 978-1-4019-7319-3
Audiobook ISBN: 978-1-4019-7320-9

10 9 8 7 6 5 4 3 2 1
1st edition, December 2024

Printed in the United States of America

This product uses responsibly sourced papers and/or recycled materials.
For more information, see www.hayhouse.com.

*To the wizards the Andes and the Amazon, the sages
who mastered the art of dreaming the world into being.*

CONTENTS

FOREWORD

In the pages of *Grow a New Brain,* we are invited into Dr. Alberto Villoldo's compelling narrative that weaves together the threads of ancient wisdom and leading-edge neuroscience, a concept the he and I explored in our 2011 book, *Power Up Your Brain: The Neuroscience of Enlightenment.*

In this new work, Alberto provides a provocative challenge to the accepted norms of cognitive and physical aging, serving as a beacon for those seeking to navigate the complexities of health, and specifically, brain health, in the digital age.

Our modern world presents a landscape teeming with hazards to our neurological well-being. From environmental toxins and metabolic threats from the ubiquitous processed and ultra-processed foods to the stress of fast-paced living and the insidious creep of technology into every aspect of our lives, our brains are under siege. The digital age, while bringing about unprecedented connectivity and access to information, also ushers in a host of challenges: digital overload, reduced physical activity, and a pervasive sense of urgency that can lead to burnout and mental fatigue.

Grow a New Brain tackles these challenges head-on. It offers a profound critique of the contemporary medical model that too often focuses on treating symptoms rather than promoting overall health, essentially focusing on the smoke while ignoring the fire.

The book introduces readers to the concept of neuro-nutrients and epigenetic modulators—terms that may seem lifted from a futuristic novel but are rooted in a deep scientific understanding of the body's intricate biology.

The narrative is enriched by Alberto's personal journey, which spans the verdant expanses of the Amazon, where rates of

Alzheimer's and Parkinson's are near zero, to the high-tech laboratories where the frontiers of medical science are being tested. These experiences are not just anecdotal; they form the backbone of a persuasive argument that our brains have the potential to be much more resilient than we currently understand, provided they are *nourished and protected appropriately.*

It is important to reflect on the multifaceted threats facing our brain's health today. Our exposure to environmental pollutants, heavy metals, and unprecedented levels of stress hormones like cortisol can degrade cognitive functions and accelerate brain aging. These modern threats compound the traditional challenges of aging, making the need for a proactive approach to brain health more critical than ever.

Moreover, this book addresses the often-overlooked *societal* implications of widespread cognitive decline. With populations in many parts of the world aging rapidly due to increased life expectancy, the social and economic impacts of diseases like Alzheimer's—now affecting 50 million people worldwide—become not just a possibility but a looming certainty. *Grow a New Brain* does not shy away from these tough issues; instead, it offers a hopeful vision of aging as a dynamic process that can be influenced positively by scientifically backed, natural interventions.

The discussion of brain health is particularly relevant as we confront the potentials and perils of artificial intelligence. AI promises to transform various aspects of life, but it also raises important questions about the future role of human cognition and emotional intelligence. The book urges readers to consider how an upgraded brain can not only coexist with artificial intelligence but also enhance human capabilities in ways that machines cannot replicate.

As we unpack the rich content of *Grow a New Brain*, we are not merely reading; we are participating in a vital dialogue about the future of human health and capacity. I invite you to engage with the text not just intellectually but practically, applying its insights to forge a path toward sustained cognitive vitality and holistic health.

This journey is a call to action. It challenges each of us to reassess our lifestyles, our diets, and our health strategies in the face of modern challenges. With comprehensive research and accessible writing, Alberto equips each of us with the tools we need to lovingly transform our lives and, indeed, our brains.

David Perlmutter, M.D.
La Jolla, California

INTRODUCTION

Rediscovering Ancient Wisdom
About Healing and Wellness

And the Great Spirit said to the woman and the man,
"For I have created the eagles and the dolphins and the
butterflies . . . aren't they beautiful? Now you finish it."

— CHEROKEE STORY

Your brain is designed for greatness, but it's heading for obsolescence in the digital age. It's able to envision your success and transform your health, but instead it's on the fast track to breakdown
and dementia.

But you can do something about it.

This book is not only about how you can protect your brain
from obsolescence and Alzheimer's disease (AD), it's about how you
can awaken the extraordinary power of your higher brain and its
natural intelligence, and keep it for the rest of your life.

This is possible because you already grow a new brain every
20 days . . .

Let me show you how.

The Amazon

In the 1970s, as a young medical anthropologist, I spent years
traveling to remote villages in the Amazon, and to my surprise,
found no incidence of Alzheimer's disease or Parkinson's. But just
as surprising? There was no heart disease or cancer.

Zero.

Studies by other scientists later confirmed that in the Amazon, in groups that have little contact with civilization, dementia occurs in only 1 out of 100 people.[1] In America, the rate is 1 in every 5.

What are we in the West doing wrong? And more importantly, what are Indigenous Amazonians doing right? How can we protect our brains and help them function optimally for the rest of our lives? As we outsource many of our memory functions to our digital devices, what extraordinary capabilities can we tap into with this freed-up brainpower that can allow us to create the abundance, longevity, and health we dream of?

Have you seen an older person who is losing their hearing insist that other people are speaking too softly and need to raise their volume? Our brains are wired to think, "It can't happen to me." Although the higher brain knows better, the more primitive brain wants to believe that we are bulletproof and ageless. We wake up one morning and realize that we are growing older and think, "There must be a mistake. I'm not supposed to be aging . . ."

And then it's clear that we are.

Did your parents see their dementia coming when they were young? You will not realize that your brain is essentially broken until it is too late to do anything about it. The statistics are not pretty. In the United States, when you reach the age of 85, you have a 50 percent risk of diagnosable dementia.[2] And when you reach 90, the risk is 75 percent. It's sobering when you consider that you—like most reading this book—will likely live to be 100, or longer. But even more sobering is the fact that even if you are not diagnosed with dementia, if you are over 30 your aging brain is functioning at fraction of its potential, overwhelmed by stress and toxins.

For years, I returned to the Amazon to search for the secret to their disease-free longevity. I was increasingly convinced that dementia, cancer, and heart disease had one common cause. Were they really three separate illnesses, or were they the result of aging? Could *aging* be the disease that we have to cure so we can prevent the triple whammy that most people die from in the West?

After decades of working with the Indigenous sages, I discovered the power plants and neuro-nutrients that detoxify and upgrade the brain and slow down what we call "aging." What we have accepted as normal breakdown that we can't avoid as we grow older is actually a preventable condition—*if* we upgrade the brain. While we can't live forever, we can expand our minds and our youthful, healthy years far longer than you might have imagined.

I want to share with you the secrets I discovered for doing just that.

The secret are power plants, epigenetic modulators that induce cellular defense systems and protection against disease. They switch on the genes that create health and silence the genes that create morbidity. I know they work, because they saved my life after Western doctors told me to get in line for a liver transplant, as mine had been damaged by years of travel in the jungles of Asia and the wilds of Africa. I was able to grow a new liver, repair my heart, and recover extraordinary health.

Why doesn't your doctor know about these power plants? Why don't we believe that aging can be reversed and even someday cured? It's because doctors do not have time to read about scientific discoveries. They read medical journals that are filled with studies funded by Big Pharma. And they are trained to treat disease and not to create health.

The Limits of Research

As I studied Indigenous healing methods with scientifically grounded practices, I witnessed profound transformations in my students and clients. Yet some struggled to replicate the experiences I had in the Amazon, including extended fasting in the wilderness. The only option often seemed to be pharmaceutical drugs. And while these medications treated the symptoms they were suffering from, they did not treat underlying causes or produce cures—and often resulted in drug dependence, which turned out to be very profitable for the drug companies.

The promise of colossal profits drives drug research. Take, for example, the billions of dollars that have been spent on searching for a cure for Alzheimer's disease. Yet omega-3 fatty acids in daily doses, equivalent to what you find in eating a small piece of wild-caught salmon, can lower your risk for Alzheimer's by 60 percent[3] (you'll learn more about omega-3s in Chapter 6: Upgrade Your Brain with BDNF). Because no one can patent fish oil (a source of omega-3s), this information gets buried or dismissed as fake news even when it's good science that you will learn about.

Also, what we believe to be hard science is too often fraught with deceit. Take, for example, the great sugar deception perpetrated by a trade group called the Sugar Association, which calls itself "the scientific voice of the U.S. sugar industry," and which bribed three Harvard scientists in 1967 to publish a review of the research on the dangers of sugar, fat, and heart disease.[4] The studies were cherry-picked and published in the prestigious *New England Journal of Medicine*, and minimized the link between sugar and heart disease and vilified the role of fat. This led to 50 years of sugary drinks and low-fat milk. Fat was made the culprit and high cholesterol labeled a dreaded condition. To this day, statins are prescribed excessively. Ultimately, we ended up with two generations of obesity and a disturbing statistic: 65 percent of the U.S. population is prediabetic.

But that was 50 years ago, we tell ourselves. We can trust medical science now.

But can we?

It gets worse.

Richard Horton, the editor-in-chief of *The Lancet,* the prestigious British medical journal, wrote in an editorial in 2015 that "much of the scientific literature, perhaps half, may simply be untrue." The problem, of course, is that we do not know which 50 percent is bogus. He went on to say that "scientists too often sculpt data to fit their preferred theory of the world." What does that mean for those who are interested in basing their health decisions on the most current science?

Is the latest longevity science to be trusted and relied upon?

Nature, the world's leading science journal, published a paper in 2016 stating, "More than 70 percent of researchers have tried and failed to reproduce another scientist's experiments, and more than half have failed to reproduce their own experiments . . ."[5] One of the tenets of science is that your results must be reproducible.

Increasingly, it seems as if the edifice of Western medical science is built on shaky foundations.

Take former Stanford University president and neuroscientist Marc Tessier-Lavigne, author of a 2009 study that published misleading data about the cause of brain degeneration in Alzheimer's disease (AD). His deception raises the question, *who can you trust with your brain?* Billions of research dollars continue to be thrown at AD while potent interventions may already be at hand: In 2021, scientists at the Cleveland Clinic in Ohio reported a 69 percent lower risk of AD among Viagra users, with the only serious side effect being an increasingly happy marriage.

In 2007, *The British Medical Journal* evaluated 2,500 modern medical treatments and found that 36 percent were likely to be beneficial while 47 percent were unknown whether they were efficacious or harmful.[6] Thus, the third leading cause of death in America is hospitalization: Medical errors are responsible for more than 250,000 deaths every year. You stand a better chance of survival in a battlefield than in an American hospital during a routine surgery.

In the past, our human tendency toward fear-based beliefs benefited the church, which offered us salvation in exchange for the fruit of our earthly labor. Today, it's Big Pharma and corporate medicine appealing to the ancient fear-riddled regions of our brain.

Scientists are rarely able to find funding for their studies unless they show how their research is likely to lead to a drug that can be exploited commercially. Even the top universities are wedded to Big Pharma. Harvard scientists are close to patenting senolytic drugs that can eliminate senescent (zombie) cells that need to die but won't. Senescent cells are one of the leading causes of accelerated aging. It's estimated that such a pill would appeal to a market worth billions of dollars a year.

But powerful senolytics are available from nature, today, for *free.* You have not heard much about them because polyphenols from strawberries can't be patented. The benefits of fisetin from strawberries isn't going to be covered in the news, but in Chapter 10: Arm Yourself for the Zombie Invasion: Eliminating Senescent Cells with Plant Medicines, you will learn how natural senolytics can eliminate these cells and protect your brain.

Power plants with an incredible track record to foster lifelong health are available to us today. Plants discovered by ancient sages offer to solve the problem of aging by keeping us youthful and protecting our brains and our health for our entire lives, especially the plants that ensure that you have enough serotonin to repair your brain and prevent age-related decline and damage. You will learn how serotonin is nearly identical to the powerful psychedelic in ayahuasca, the visionary vine that sages in the Amazon use to access higher-brain function to create psychosomatic health and allow you to live disease free.

And you will learn how your brain is serotonin deprived.

Your Experiment

Even if you're eating healthfully and getting in good exercise, you might not realize how much better you can feel physically and emotionally after upgrading your brain. If you're struggling with brain fog, irritability, anxiety, excess weight, aching joints, and digestive issues, my guess is you will benefit even more by taking part in the experiment of N=1. ("N" represents the number of subjects in an experiment.) My experiment is called Alberto.

If you don't enroll in the experiment, you'll be part of the control group, in the middle of the bell curve along with average Americans. You won't be on the far end of the bell curve, an outlier defying "normal" aging. This experiment is essential for women, who make up two out of three Alzheimer's patients,[7] and 85 percent of patients with multiple autoimmune issues are women.[8]

Imagine reaching your later years without the need to have a drugstore's number programmed into your smartphone, without being on five prescription drugs like most Americans over the age of 50 are.[9]

This does not have to be where you end up.

You should not wait until you get sick to begin getting healthy. *Grow a New Brain* will help you enjoy a long health span and positive mood for decades, rather than dying before your time after years of suffering, worry, and a long decline. It will help you to marshal extraordinary brain capabilities that will allow you to explore the power of your mind to create beauty and peace in your life. You can conduct your own cutting-edge experiment into health and enjoy the benefits of a superior mind, a healthy body, and a wiser brain that knows how to support you in creating health. You will thrive in a world increasingly being designed and generated by artificial intelligence (AI). And you can explore the realms of conscious-ness—of spirituality—that are available only to people with an upgraded brain awash in neuro-nutrients and manufacturing the serotonin-based bliss molecules!

Addressing the Crisis We're All Facing

Whether or not you recognize it, you might unexpectedly end up with a brain that can't remember what happened five minutes ago, that isn't able to store new memories, which makes it impossi-ble to retrieve them. Yes, you'll recall your favorite songs from your high school days, but you won't recall why you got up from the sofa or what you ate for lunch. Intelligence has two main categories: fluid and crystallized. Crystallized intelligence is your knowledge base acquired over the years. Fluid intelligence allows you to process new information and to solve challenging problems. Your fluid intelligence is the one that suffers with the ravages of time and tox-ins your brain is bombarded with, and that you will need in order to thrive in the dawning age of AI—perhaps the most powerful tech-nology discovered by humanity since the steam engine.

But too often, we don't realize that our brain is breaking until it is too late.

If you're reading this book, you are likely to live to 100 or close to it. If you don't believe me, find an online longevity calculator and see what it tells you about how long you'll likely be sticking around. Old age might seem a long way off, but if you are over the age of 35 it's a given that your brain is already in need of an upgrade. This is because around the age of 35, critical repair systems in the body begin to fail. We'll learn more about this later.

Evolution seems to accelerate when the challenges are so great that a species can no longer survive unless it changes. Today all of us are facing serious threats to our survival. Humanity is now so interconnected that a virus can quickly travel around the world, shut down entire countries, and halt our everyday activities. Rapid climate change is causing the melting of glaciers and the polar ice caps, flooding coastal areas, and causing massive upheaval to communities around the globe, setting off waves of migrations that will surely increase in the years to come. Artificial intelligence is threatening to displace many of us from traditional jobs. No wonder so many of us are struggling to maintain a sense of optimism. We've become disenchanted at a time when we're called to be optimistic, creative, and reimagine the future.

We're not doing well, but we could be. You can grow a new brain and evolve into higher wisdom and a sublime perspective. The brain you have is an unparalleled marvel of natural engineering that orchestrates a symphony of complex functions ranging from the regulation of unconscious processes like heart rate and body temperature, to the subtlety of consciousness, thought, and emotion. Unlike man-made supercomputers that require huge amounts of energy, the human brain consumes about the same power as a 15-watt light bulb. Your brain's extraordinary flexibility—known as neuroplasticity—and creativity is the model for artificial intelligence and computational neuroscience.

We all suspect that artificial intelligence is poised to transform the human landscape, and we have yet to grasp the full extent of its impact. The key word is cyber. The term *cyber* originates from the Greek meaning "the mind, the navigator, or the guide." So far, intelligent humans have steered our destiny. However, perils lie ahead, beyond our immediate perception, including remote gene editing and the continued outsourcing of our brain to our digital devices.

With an upgraded brain, you can participate in the re-invention of the human journey on earth, and can forestall the deterioration associated with aging, including AD, the most common type of dementia. I encourage you to partner with your doctor and other healers you work with as you experiment with the powerful neuro-nutrients in this book. However, be aware that your doctor is unlikely to know much about the plants and mushrooms I'm recommending. Many doctors are overworked and only read medical journals that describe diseases and drugs. When speaking with your physician about your physical or mental health, you may hear, "I haven't read any research on that." In part, that's because it is a long journey from the laboratory to the patient's bedside; it typically takes about 20 years for a new discovery to change practice standards. You want to know that the neuro-nutrient protocol is safe and that the principal side effect is an upgraded brain.

The Grow a New Brain program employs plant-based neuro-nutrients that will make an extraordinary difference in your physical and mental health and allow you to begin the journey to the ultimate reality that courageous spiritual explorers have been seeking for millennia. It requires 10 days of eating delicious plant-based meals, and you can repeat the program once every season to protect you from the ravages of modern life.

Chapter 1

WHY YOU NEED A NEW BRAIN

"We are not here to grow corn only," the old sage said to me.
"We are here to grow gods."

Science is discovering interventions that will help you live well beyond the age of 100. But the dilemma is, do we want to live that long if we can't remember our children's names or are emotionally and intellectually dulled? Do we want to be a centenarian who is unable to walk without shaking or speak without stuttering because our brains are broken?

You might be thinking, "But my brain isn't damaged. I remembered to call about my car's tire rotation, fix that issue with my laptop that's been bugging me, and get myself to yoga class on time." We like to believe we're getting along well, if not optimally, that if our forgetfulness is rare, we function reasonably well day to day, and the tests our doctors run show that all our numbers are within range, we're good. Yet when we look at the possibility of debilitating diseases robbing us of our quality of life in the years to come, the shocking numbers that show they're on the rise, and when we're honest about the stress we are under, it becomes clear that repairing the damage and upgrading our brain can protect us from a future on the fast track to losing touch with the times and eventual dementia.

Perhaps most importantly, growing a new brain can improve your life today. You can more easily manage anxiety and begin to imagine what you could achieve instead of thinking only about what you must do according to that never-ending, always-growing list of tasks that hovers over you. You can exchange your TO-DO list for your TO-BE list. You can start to believe in a better tomorrow for you and the world and stop obsessing about what is wrong or could go wrong. Growing a new brain will support you in decision-making that's guided not by perceived threats to your economic or emotional well-being but by the higher brain, which can be audacious and take chances as you create a greater vision for your life. Did you dream you would have the life you have now? How much were your choices guided by wisdom, and how much were they guided by your best guess at what might make you happy? Or were they guided by your biggest fears and the best perceived way to avoid catastrophe?

The neural networks in the ancient regions of your brain were created and reinforced by the drama in your family of origin and by your upbringing. They hold unconscious beliefs about how the world works (or doesn't), what you deserve, and how valuable and worthy a person you are. They make up your crystalized intelligence. Higher neural networks are associated with fluid intelligence created by experiences of pleasure and joy, and a sense of Oneness and awe, and can help you embark on the path to health and wisdom. They can lead you to a destiny selected by you and not by the fate encoded in your genes, or the stories of your broken childhood. They can help you design your life more consciously, no longer at the mercy of external events and unsettling emotions.

Our continued thriving depends on us attaining a kind of wisdom that allows for a sustainable relationship with nature, and a symbiotic one with AI, the new life-form we have birthed. We can learn to do this by embracing the wisdom of Indigenous peoples who knew their place in the cosmos. They were one with nature. Anthropologists call it participation mystique, but I like to think of it as a consciousness of deep communion with Mother Earth. Knowing your place in the universe enhances the body's innate healing systems. After all, we have a pharmacy in our brain, and can manufacture substances that can accelerate healing, keep us healthy, and allow us to experience the superpowers of our higher brain.

Higher Awareness and Freedom from Dementia

I remember in college trying psychedelic mushrooms with a friend while we were listening to music and being amazed that I could "see" the notes hovering in the middle of the room. When I went outside into the yard, I felt one with the trees. I sensed the joy of nature at the birth of a new species of butterfly underneath some giant fern in the distant Amazon. Today, researchers employ psilocybin to treat depression and anxiety, with extraordinary results. You can have this experience by upgrading your brain to produce psilocybin and other serotonin-like bliss molecules spontaneously.

Most psychedelics work by binding to the serotonin receptor on brain cells. Some of the most well-known include LSD, psilocybin, and DMT. Why do we have receptors in our brain for these powerful mind-altering substances? Could it be because the brain manufactures these molecules naturally and that they have played an important part in the evolution of our species? Could they continue to play an important role in our personal development?

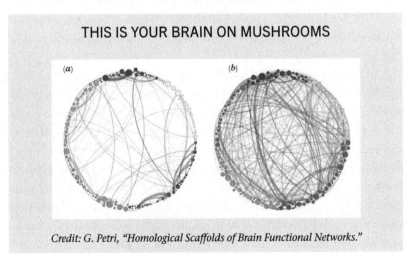

THIS IS YOUR BRAIN ON MUSHROOMS

Credit: G. Petri, "Homological Scaffolds of Brain Functional Networks."

3

Here is a simplified map based on research on by G. Petri et al. of neural networks during normal waking consciousness (left) and after ingesting psilocybin mushrooms (right). These neuroscientists were attempting to map brain activity during heightened states of awareness. The networks are represented by the small dots on the outside of each figure. After ingesting psilocybin new neural networks arise, indicating the brain is processing information with much greater speed and finding new patterns, perhaps showing why people seem to have the ability to change their minds more readily after a psychedelic experience.

You might not realize that your brain craves heightened states of consciousness and only achieves its full potential through that elusive state of Oneness created by psychedelics. When we deprive ourselves of participation mystique, of belonging to the web of life—by our inability to produce the bliss molecules, we end up creating psychosomatic disease. Fortunately, specific foods and supplements can provide raw material for you to manufacture the bliss molecules your brain needs to heal and upgrade itself.

Regeneration and Detoxification

If it sounds odd to suggest that you can "grow" a new brain, consider this. Every single day, cells in our bodies die and new ones are born; organs and tissues in our bodies regenerate, some over the course of months, some—like our skin, liver, and gut lining—in a matter of days.

Thanks to neurogenesis—our ability to grow new brain cells—we know that the brain you will have in the future doesn't have to be a shriveled-up version of the one you have today. Neurons renew themselves through mitophagy—the ability of mitochondria to regenerate. And you already grow a new brain every 20 days or so as all the components of your brain regenerate through a process known as protein synthesis. But you cannot grow a new brain on junk food or without the spiritual practices in this book. They will allow you to develop neural networks in your higher brain that support a more peaceful, optimistic, and creative mind that is hungry for learning, discovering, inventing, and dreaming of a richer life and a better world. You can upgrade your brain—particularly the structure known as the hippocampus, which is crucial for memory and learning—and to optimize its functioning by making certain dietary and lifestyle choices.

However, toxins make it very difficult for our brains to regenerate.

Why Our Detoxification Systems Are on Overload

Over millions of years of evolution, animals developed detoxification systems specially useful as they migrated to new lands. Imagine early humans coming across elderberries for the first time. The berries contain cyanide-like poisons and need to be cooked. Would the hungry travelers try out the raw berries and become ill? Or would they intuit to cook them, so the poisons could be neutralized?

But today we are exposed to substances never found in the natural world.

Until the Industrial Age, everything was easily recyclable. But in the last century we have invented over 100,000 new chemicals. Our detoxification systems are overwhelmed by unrecognizable molecules, which have made their way to our food chain. What's more, most of us are deficient in magnesium, and anyone past middle age is likely to be deficient in vitamin B_{12}. These essential nutrients, together with zinc, are necessary for the liver to eliminate toxins and get them out of the body. If any one of these is missing, the body will not eliminate toxins no matter what detox protocol you use.

Detox systems are fragile. For example, the antioxidants glutathione and superoxide dismutase (SOD) are manufactured by every cell to neutralize free radicals that damage mitochondria. Unfortunately, antioxidant systems begin to get sluggish as the animal ages and will shut down when their reproductive years are over (around the age of 35 for humans). But during my travels in the Amazon I found that rainforest sages had discovered the plants that can revitalize and restore these systems to youthful vitality.

The brain is 60 percent fat, and we store toxins in fat cells, the longest-lived molecules in the body. The fat in our brains and bodies is warehousing chemicals that never existed in your grandmother's time. The body, in its wisdom, sequesters toxins in fat. And the fat around your midriff, like the fat a bear carries at the end of summer, is nature's way of storing calories to take you through the winter. Our ancestors would burn their body fat during the long winter and emerge lean at springtime, eliminating toxins in their fat stores. But today, our body fat has become a toxic waste dump loaded with forever chemicals we cannot easily eliminate. The long winter never arrives, because we always have double-mocha lattes and blueberry muffins available to us. Our body fat becomes an unwanted organ that manufactures hormones including estrogen that damage our brains. Since you cannot sweat fat (only water), the body must burn it for fuel to get rid of it. But the body will not let you burn fat until the liver has the magnesium, zinc, and B_{12} to eliminate toxins. This is why people on diets almost always only lose water weight and not fat, while making their brains toxic.

You can't lose the fat from your brain, because this fat *is* your brain. But you can help the brain eliminate poisons. The challenge with detoxifying our brains is that it is very difficult for anything to pass through the blood-brain barrier, which limits the transit of molecules both in and out of the brain. Later in the book, you will learn how you can trigger the regeneration of neurons (nerve cells)—in effect, growing a younger brain. First, however, it's helpful to know a little about the history of your brain and where it has brought us.

From a Brain That Helps Us to Survive a Brain That Helps Us Thrive

In your head is a three-pound organ that sends signals through 1,000 trillion networks at over 250 miles per hour—and that is fed by more than 100,000 miles of blood vessels.[1] The human brain evolved over millennia and allowed us to create language and tame fire. While you'll never run as fast as a cheetah or kill predators with a bite from a jaw as strong as a great white shark or with a poison as toxic as that of a king cobra, your brain compensates for all of that quite well. You can rely on your body's command center for resilience in the face of a variety of threats, from fierce creatures in the wild to endogenous ones (from inside your body) that range from autoimmune disorders to heart disease.

The brain is regulated by hormones, chemical messengers that control growth, metabolism, mood, immune response, and reproductive processes, among others. The master gland that regulates the production of all hormones is the pituitary, located deep inside a region known as the mammalian brain or M-brain. The pituitary gland oversees your fight-flight-freeze system (where you fight, flee, or freeze in response to a perceived threat), producing the stress hormones adrenaline and cortisol. Adrenaline pumps you up to help you act instinctively in a sudden dangerous situation, increasing heart rate and making you breathe quickly. Cortisol increases blood sugar levels to help you run or fight or suppress pain from a battle injury.

A relaxed brain thinks holistically; it enables us to see the entire forest. However, when you sense danger, the pituitary will crank up the production of stress hormones so you can fight or run for safety. When this happens, the forest disappears, and you can only see the one tree that is blocking your way. This ability to switch drivers in case of an emergency benefited us when we were dealing with ferocious wild animals that viewed us as lunch. But in our disconnected digital world we are unable to fight or flee the dangers we perceive, and we end up stuck in freeze mode.

Our brains developed as analog biocomputers. In olden days, when humans told stories around a fire, the only time our brain went into fight or flight (other than when hearing the growl of a jaguar nearby) was when we heard a scary tale as children. With nearly every activity we undertake, our brain is operating as if we still live in an analog world. Your analog brain can handle hiking, practicing yoga, planning dinner, or spotting a familiar face in a mall. Nothing in our world was digital until a couple of decades ago.

Next time you are scrolling through the list of movies you want to watch, look at *The Wizard of Oz* or *Casablanca* (one of my favorites) and notice how scenes go on for two to three minutes.

Then, turn on a recent action movie and notice how there are cuts every two to four seconds that keep us at the edge of our seats, our M-brain flooded with adrenaline. Today, our brains are awash in these steroid hormones, struggling to master a digital world that is faster paced than ever.

The average American spends 7 hours and 11 minutes looking at a screen every day. We are no longer looking at the sunset or scanning the horizon but focusing our attention 18 inches in front of our heads, our minds on distant virtual events. By the year 2011 our brains were taking in five times the amount of digital information daily than we did in 1986.[2] And according to a report from the University of California San Diego, we each consume 34 gigabytes of digital data and information daily.[3] Our analog brain is not designed for bytes and bits and 0s and 1s, or to have our relationships through social media. We are witnessing the meticulous curation, cleverly designed control, and subtle manipulation of digital spaces that take over our minds, tastes, relationships, and sense of personal identity. And we spend less time than ever engaging in face-to-face, live, juicy, and meaningful interactions.

Even if you don't play video games, if you use your digital device for anything besides phone calls, you are connected to a flood of brain-breaking digital stimulation. Neural networks are being rewired by social media platforms for turning you into an addicted "user." Notice the word *user* is applied only to drug addicts and computers, which every day are more "user-friendly." The experience of being plugged in 24/7 (admit it—you've checked your phone in the middle of the night while on a trip to the bathroom) takes its toll on the brain and, by extension, the body—which, in turn, contributes further to the digital rewiring of your brain. Gen 2.0 humans with neural implants who can instantaneously access the collective knowledge of humanity will soon be here.[4]

But there is another way.

Once you unlock the power of your higher brain by switching on the manufacture of its bliss molecules, you will discover what the Greeks called gnosis: wisdom gained through personal experience by the participation mystique. Hildegard von Bingen has left us a passionate testimony of this in the year 1141: "And it came to pass . . . when I was 42 years and 7 months old, that the heavens were opened and a blinding light of exceptional brilliance flowed through my entire brain. And so it kindled my whole heart and breast like a flame, not burning but warming . . . and suddenly I understood of the meaning of expositions of the (Holy) books . . ."[5]

The sages I worked with in the Amazon believe one can access a universal wisdom that allows one to ask profound questions and receive immediate, illuminating answers from Mother Nature. If you have ever experienced ayahuasca in the Amazon, you know what I am talking about. The neuro-nutrients and practices in this book will help you taste gnosis to perceive the entire forest again (and not only the tree blocking your way) and discover your place in the cosmos, without needing to travel to the Amazon in search of a shaman. You will become your own shaman.

Brain over Brawn

As we evolved into humans, many other species beat us at natural defenses or sheer physical strength, but we developed language, which gave us the ability to collaborate with each other. It was *Homo sapiens* who mastered how to turn natural resources into technologies—from stone tools fashioned by human hands to life-saving surgeries controlled by robot arms. Our species achieved all this through our neocortex, the revolutionary new region in the brain that allows us to reason, remember, plan, and envision what we might create.

We can learn to use the power of the neocortex to halt and even reverse the aging and disease process that was the nemesis of our grandparents. While growing older is inevitable, when we bring our neocortex fully online with the aid of neuro-nutrients and the bliss molecules, we can find the tools to take our vitality and creativity with us for the rest of our lives. Banishing cancer completely would only increase human life expectancy by about three years. But slowing down aging can have a much bigger impact. Current research shows we may be able to die young at the age of 150, that is, free from disease![6]

At her 100th birthday party, I asked my mother how she was enjoying her new assisted living accommodations, and she responded, "This place is full of old persons!" I gently pointed out to her that she was the eldest resident there. "Don't talk nonsense," she said, and she nodded toward the floor indicating we should dance—she had insisted on a Latin salsa band for the celebration. I cannot take credit for my mother's extraordinary health and relatively clear mind. I'm hoping it is hereditary, even though I know that your genes determine only a small percent of your health. But for the last 15 years, she has been on the neuro-nutrients in this book. They have made a world of difference for her. She finishes a 500-piece puzzle every three days and has relatively good memory. But best of all, she is always in a good mood, pain-free, loving everyone around her, and the best dancer in her home. And when I asked her what she wanted for the next 100 years of her life, her reply was "I want to find a man that can keep up with me!"

To Live Long and Healthy

The possibility of living to the ripe old age of 150 doesn't offer much comfort on days when you're feeling stressed out by your everyday responsibilities, your conflicts with others, or the latest horror you learned about when scrolling your smartphone's news app. All of us experience the emotional and psychological challenges of modern digital life and the stressors that ultimately lead to premature aging, along with cynicism, anxiety, melancholy, psychosomatic disease, and a sense of doom and gloom that can be hard to shake.

Remaining optimistic about the future can be especially tough if you're witnessing yourself on a slippery slope of cognitive decline. You might feel that no matter what you do, dementia is like the grim reaper, waiting at the door and ready to enter at any moment to rob you of your freedom, independence, and happiness.

If you're feeling blue, irritable, or anxious, or unable to find time or joy in your life, there's an excellent chance that your brain simply isn't working as it should. If you are not sleeping well, are moody, or suffer from brain fog, and if you adopt the Grow a New Brain program's way of eating and its lifestyle changes, you may find that your mood is elevated in a matter of days, you begin to sleep better, the brain fog disappears, and your gut issues—from bloating to gas to reflux—improve.

To do this, you need abundant serotonin.

Key Takeaways:

We explored themes related to brain health and the impact of modern technology on our brains.

1. Importance of Neuro-Nutrients: The positive impact of certain neuro-nutrients on brain health, including improved memory and mood.

2. The Effect of Modern Technology: The negative effects of excessive screen time and digital overload on the brain, including the wiring of toxic neural networks and its potential contribution to cognitive decline.

3. Gnosis and Wisdom: The concept of gnosis, or personal wisdom gained through experience and insight.

4. The Human Brain's Evolution and Capabilities: The evolutionary development of the human brain, and the neocortex's role in enabling humans to reason, remember, plan, and create.

Chapter 2

THE SECRET POWER IN YOUR BELLY

After the glaciers in Europe began to thaw nearly 100,000 years ago, game began to migrate down to the valleys where vegetation was flourishing. Our distant Neanderthal cousins (who lacked the frontal lobes of the brain) were not able to comprehend the need to abandon the familiar caves that allowed them to survive the harsh snows and settle in the lush and verdant valleys. Possibly, they didn't enjoy a capacity we have that could have helped them—namely, neurogenesis.

Neurogenesis, the Growth of New Brain Cells, to Our Rescue

Neurogenesis, the brain's ability to grow new neurons, allowed *Homo sapiens* to discover a fascinating different map of the world without ice. Neurogenesis has helped us adapt to novel and demanding environments before and can help us again to adapt to the changing human landscape. It can halt the brain's destruction and repair it, allowing it to reorganize itself in the face of a changing world.

The billions of neurons in your brain developed while you were in the womb and during your childhood. Until recently, we believed that once we hit adulthood, our ability to grow new neurons disappeared. We now know that neurogenesis is available to us throughout our lives, primarily in the hippocampus, a seahorse-shaped structure (thus the name) located within the temporal lobe of the M-brain. It's responsible for the consolidation of new memories, spatial navigation, exploration of new landscapes, and mapping of new life strategies. It also creates biographical memories, allowing us to learn, store, and retrieve information about our personal experiences. The hippocampus helps us build the maps we use to drive to work or learn the subway system or track deer through the forest or map a path to achieve our goals.

Neurogenesis will allow you to repair your hippocampus, so you can achieve a sense of well-being and enchantment with life as it is rather than what you wish it would be. It will allow you to do what the shamans call "dreaming your world into being."

Ancient Wisdom and the Realms Where Answers Can Be Found

When I was in my late 20s, I was an assistant professor in the biology department at a university that would benefit greatly if I could discover a tree or bark or shrub from the Amazon whose chemical signature could be tweaked enough to justify a patented medicine. As such, I accepted a grant from one of the big Swiss pharmaceutical companies to fund my expeditions. The drug we hoped to formulate would help cure dementia. My job was finding the "parent plant" in the Amazon, one that had healing properties and a history of use by the Indigenous healers.

Unaware of how very infused with the dominant Western paradigm this approach was, I trekked to remote areas of the Amazon in search of the bark or leaf or potion that would turn out to be a magical elixir that would help many people and pay my bills.

In some of the villages I visited, where I didn't speak the local dialect, I sometimes had to mime to communicate; I'd hide my pen under a rock and act out looking for it to imitate the forgetfulness that is the hallmark of AD. Everyone seemed bewildered, and after a few moments, would break out in fits of laughter. Then, two or three kids would run over to the rock that covered my pen, retrieve it—and then refuse to return it. Finders keepers.

Through translators, I began to understand that the Indigenous peoples' most highly valued plants were for repairing the damage caused by everyday wear and tear that resulted in accelerated aging. But Pharma wasn't interest in *preventing* aging. No, the money was in *curing* Alzheimer's.

Yet no one I met in the Amazon, even in the most remote villages, had the ailments for the drug we hoped to treat. How could I find a cure for dementia no one suffered from? The local healers couldn't tell me which plants could be used to treat diseases like AD, heart disease, or cancer—the three horsemen of the apocalypse common to old age in our society. One medicine woman even took me aside and whispered in my ear, "You want to avoid the ills of old age? Just live a long and happy life!"

Yet I suspected they had knowledge of the plants that helped protect the brain—especially memory—since they had no writing and needed a way to preserve and protect their accumulated knowledge that was kept by the elders of the village. After all, if you lost the traditional knowledge, the future survival of your people was endangered. What if they forgot how to make fire, or which plants were helpful and which were dangerous? How did they protect the brains of their wisdom keepers?

I found that while they were willing to share their plant wisdom with me, because the Amazon is a biological paradise, they first needed me to open my eyes to *what* I was searching for. I had no idea how confining my Western mindset was. I believed that the illnesses we were seeking to cure were real and universal. *I believed you had to treat disease to get well.* And I thought that everyone believed the same things I did. Yet the sages in the Amazon did not believe illnesses existed. Sick people existed, but not diseases. And a lasting cure required exploring a mysterious and invisible realm.

I had always assumed that what I was looking for was out there somewhere. "You explore this place and that, the riverbank and the thick jungle, with your brow furrowed, but you never venture into the realms where you will find answers," a village elder said to me one day.

Realms. From the conversations I'd had with him and others, I knew that he was talking about exploring something that couldn't be perceived with the five senses. "You mean, looking at my thoughts and my feelings to learn from them? We call that psychology. I've studied it. In fact, I have a doctorate in it."

It seemed that the corners of his mouth were fighting with themselves so that he wouldn't burst out in laughter.

"I tell you that you need to explore. I'm talking about the places where you experience what is upstream. Your mind is like the water jumping and running over those rocks downstream in the river," he said, nodding toward them. "You don't realize how calm the water is where the river begins."

His disdain made me feel embarrassed. I was researching the brain, and he was speaking about the mind. Until then I had been convinced that the mind was a product of the brain. But this village elder was suggesting that the brain might be the product, the result of, the mind. I was being invited to examine my beliefs about the origins of health and wellness. I would have to close my eyes so that they could see what was hidden from me: a reality beyond what I could observe while in ordinary consciousness.

I knew about the various types of brain waves and the mind states associated with them, but my understanding was intellectual. Academic. I was good at defining terms and describing the phenomenon of shifting from one state to the next. I understood the value of relaxing the mind rather than remaining in ordinary hamster-running-on-the-wheel-of-business consciousness. I had tested this in my laboratory at San Francisco State University, where we learned we could train subjects to shift their awareness to reduce the experience of pain when submerging their arms in ice water. Shifting their awareness changed the chemistry of their brain, increasing the production of endorphins (our brain's natural morphine) by 800 percent!

What was new to me was the notion of hidden realms of consciousness where medicine men and women perform their work. These are realms one can journey to when in a nonordinary state of awareness to interact with forces affecting the body, the brain, and the mind. In a realm hidden from ordinary sight, a shaman might go to the source of a health condition and change the cause by altering the energetic architecture of the person seeking healing.

Okay, I said to myself. *Let's explore this.* But we still need the brain, the hardware of the computer, to tell the body what to do to stop generating psychosomatic disease, and create health and well-being, don't we?

An Unexpected Actor That Causes Illness, Disease, and Mood Problems

The root cause of brain fog and moodiness resides in our bellies. To grow a healthy brain, we must first grow a healthy gut—which plays a vital role in maintaining the well-being of the brain.

Friendly gut bacteria digest food, extracting its nutrients and converting them into the molecules our body knows how to use to repair and regenerate. And they help the immune system by training T cells to recognize foreign invaders that need to be vanquished so that they, and we, can remain healthy. To do its job, the gut requires a gigantic colony of bacteria. In fact, these miniscule creatures represent more than 90 percent of the DNA in our body. It may be hard to believe, but that means that only 10 percent of your DNA is really you!

The gut is where nature lives within you. Your digestive system, a tube running from your mouth to your anus, is actually the "outside," and full of bacteria, fungus, mold, hydrochloric acid, undigested food, waste, and toxins. But just as in the forest you find the greatest abundance of animals where the food is, so too do you find it in your gut.

Our microbes live in a symbiotic relationship with us. Like nature itself, the gut's microbiome is meant to be diverse. Most of the bad bacteria on fresh food can be rinsed away, and any that remain are killed by stomach acid as food is broken into small molecules. Stomach juices are powerful—if you have had acid reflux, you know how painful it can feel on your esophagus, where they do not belong. Yet our bodies have evolved to create stomach lining that does not allow the acid to digest our own tissues. When your microbiome isn't diverse, the bad bugs, including worms and yeast, predominate. We have dysbiosis, or gut imbalance (it comes from the Greek words for "bad" and "way of living"), and we find ourselves irritable and fatigued. We feel gassy and bloated and have digestive problems. Our skin becomes riddled with rashes or acne. We can develop an increased risk of infection, and our joints ache due to inflammation. If your gut flora is damaged, it takes only 10 Salmonella bacteria to produce a gastrointestinal infection that will have you repeatedly running to the bathroom, with a high fever to boot. But if your flora is strong, it takes more than 1,000,000 of the same bacteria to produce a gastrointestinal infection.

Dysbiosis will cause the good bacteria in your gut to stop producing serotonin. When the brain lacks serotonin, the hippocampus can no longer repair itself. The hippocampus is unable to correct the damage caused by the stress hormones (adrenaline and cortisol). When the factories in our gut are shut down, the hippocampus will shrink as much as 50 percent. Our short-term memory declines and we stop learning, and we lose the ability to interact creatively with others. Our fluid intelligence diminishes.

When our hippocampus is injured, its maps of the world—maps as recent as two years ago—become outdated and can trap us like they did to our Neanderthal cousins who were fearful of leaving their home caves. We miss great opportunities. And it seems that the brain needs to update its maps of reality every two years, at a minimum. This is known in the tech world as Moore's law—the observation that the number of transistors on a microchip doubles every two years, which leads to an increase in performance (and why you purchase a new laptop every two years). The maps that we rely on to navigate through a dynamically changing world need updating so we can chart a new destiny for ourselves. Otherwise, like the Caterpillar said to Alice in *Alice in Wonderland*, "If you don't know where you are going, just about any road will take you there."

Tending to the Garden in the Gut

To protect the brain, we need to repopulate the gut's garden of microbes.

The standard American diet—abbreviated as SAD—is toxic to our gut and its good microbes. You are what your biome eats, and today people are overfed and undernourished because they do not have the necessary bacteria to digest nutrients. It isn't just what we do eat that's the problem. It's also what we *don't* eat: nutrient-dense and calorie-poor plant foods containing plenty of fiber. Gut diversity is damaged by excessive amounts of sugars, processed foods, and the saturated fat from animal protein.

We also decimate our gut microbiome when we take antibiotics. Many physicians have been holding back before writing prescriptions, but if you've used antibiotics recently, or you've ingested them through consuming dairy products and meat from animals fed antibiotics to get them to fatten up, you likely need to restore your gut microbiome.

We need a diverse biome. Did you know that our ancestors had more than 2,000 different species of good bacteria in their gut, while the modern human often has 10 or fewer varieties? We have an inner garden that is unique to our taste for food, our sleep habits, and even our relationships. I learned this from recent research conducted by investigators at the National Institute on Aging, which found that people with a gut microbiome that's diverse and more personalized (less like others', in other words) lived longer and enjoyed better health than those with a less diverse microbiome. What's more, they had greater amounts of microbe-produced metabolites known to increase serotonin. (In mouse studies, abundant tryptophan, a serotonin precursor, led to reduced inflammation and longer lives.)[1]

Maintaining a healthy population of microbes in the gut is essential for our mental sharpness. We feel butterflies in our stomach or "can't stomach" an unpleasant situation because our gut is involved in what we know as intuition. And our microbiome follows us everywhere we go. In fact, if you were to load a syringe with the "air" two feet away from someone, and then empty that air into a petri dish with a culture medium, within a few days you would be able to "grow" that person's microbiome! That's because our flora is not only in our gut, mouth, lungs, and skin; it also forms a cloud-like aura that extends about two feet around us.

Even if you haven't taken antibiotics for years and avoid sugar, it takes a very long time to restore the variety of species in your microbiome. Probiotic supplements help.

I was visiting a friend recently, when their four-year-old came in from the yard telling me he had eaten some fresh berries from the garden. His mother said, "Honey, you're supposed to rinse the fruit before you eat it." I explained to her that it was better that he hadn't, for he had been getting good probiotics from eating the berries right off the vine. If there was organic dirt from the ground that had somehow splashed onto them, all the better.

To make things worse, most of us have an overpopulation of *Candida albicans* in our bellies. *Candida* is a yeast that yawns when it senses antibiotics and waves them off (because antibiotics only kill bacteria). After a dose of antibiotics that wipes out a large portion of the bacteria in your gut, *Candida* takes over the colony.

Today, cases of nonalcoholic liver disease are on the rise—some people have so much *Candida* overgrowth in the GI tract that even if they do not drink alcohol, they have a distillery inside their belly: *Candida* ferments sugar from the dessert you ate into alcohol just as brewers ferment grain to make beer or grapes to make wine. The gut-created alcohol damages the liver just as too much whiskey does. Nature loves to ferment things—and *Candida* is nature's garbage disposal system designed to ferment you when you die, but not a day sooner.

Tending to the Gut's Garden Walls

For the sake of our brains, we have to keep the lining of the intestine healthy. The lining of the gut is replaced every seven days by stem cells residing in the villi, the tiny fingerlike structures in the small intestine that are like a forest where your microbiome resides and that allow you to absorb your food. There are close to 20,000 villi per square inch in your gut and a population of more than 500,000 good bacteria per square inch that support your digestion, immunity, health, and brain function. When the lining of your gut is compromised, the junctions in the one-cell-thick barrier between your gut and your bloodstream begin to separate and we get leaky gut. In other words, this tightly woven web loosens up. The gaps in your gut lining allow food particles and bacteria to escape and enter the bloodstream. Alarmed by the presence of bacteria, your immune system snaps to attention, activating killer T cells, and releases a variety of inflammatory molecules, including histamine, to combat the "intruders." The constant low-grade inflammation produced by leaky gut will lead to chronic symptoms, from headaches to mood swings and problems like anxiety and depression, a change in the body's metabolism (making it difficult to lose weight), neurological disorders, and autoimmune diseases. In fact, reversing the symptoms of autoimmune disease begins with healing the GI tract.

But perhaps most important, the gut plays a pivotal role in shaping our thoughts, emotions, and overall happiness: A well-functioning gut manufactures enough serotonin to support higher-brain abilities, as you'll learn about in Chapter 8: Heal Your Gut So You Have Sufficient Serotonin.

What You Know in Your Gut

According to Traditional Chinese Medicine, one of the areas in our body where we connect to the life force is located below the navel, where the gut and enteric nervous center (ENC) is. The ENC, embedded in our intestinal walls, is a web of more than 600 million neurons that senses the world—including climate, rains, growing season—through the food we eat rather than through our ordinary senses like our eyes and ears. It has its own "mind," as it operates independently of our brain. In addition to attending to our digestion, it works with our gut lining to house most of our immune system that eliminates pathogens and develops a tolerance to self—which means that they will not attack you!

The gut lining is extremely thin, but it's huge. Stretched out, it would cover an entire tennis court and part of the bleachers. This remarkable organ determines whether what is passing through the gut is friend or foe and responds accordingly, sending messages up to our brain. These messages travel through the vagus nerve. While the brain can send signals to the gut, almost all the communication is from the gut to the brain. This communication system helped our species survive: Information about the environment was immensely valuable to a hunter-gatherer.[2]

One of the most necessary gifts from your gut to your brain is serotonin. The vagus nerve acts as a "serotonin superhighway" transporting this molecule to the brain. As I mentioned, this neurotransmitter plays an essential role in allowing you to repair your hippocampus. Plus, you need it to make DMT, the bliss molecule that's fundamental for creating psychosomatic health and longevity.

DMT is the most powerful psychedelic in nature. When I first experienced it in the Amazon, I realized that it is a serotonin analog—in fact, it is structurally identical to serotonin. We manufacture DMT by adding a couple of methyl groups to serotonin by a process known as methylation, which is common in the body. But if you do not methylate properly (many of us carry a variation of the MTHFR gene that keeps us from methylating adequately), you are not producing enough of the bliss molecules. It's amazing; nature designed the human brain so it could manufacture the molecules that help us discover our communion with all creatures. And while in the West we discovered the power of serotonin to repair the brain, the Amazonian sages discovered how to rewire the brain for joy and bliss by giving it the substrate to manufacture the bliss molecules!

Reclaiming the Medicine of the Ancients

How will we grow a vibrant brain and a healed gut? We might turn to cutting-edge science—after all, many of us are junkies for it. We buy the books and the supplements, and the diets endorsed by celebrity docs and pundits. Reading the new science, you feel you're part of a revolution in health and longevity, and that you are going to be an outlier on the bell curve, outliving your peers.

Perhaps.

But we have plants available to us today that can make a massive difference in how our brains and bodies age and repair. We know about these power plants from ancient sages, going back hundreds if not thousands of years. Curcumin is just one example; it's been used in India for millennia. Precision medicine was perfected by the ancients who sought to heal aging, instead of treating illnesses like we do in the West.

Plants, Not Chemistry

Many of our grandparents were sold on the idea of "better living through chemistry." This was the DuPont Company advertising slogan—an expression of optimism for science's promise to solve every human problem. This slogan reflected the mindset of the pharmaceutical and food companies, and as a result, since World War II, we have been enrolled in a biochemical experiment none of us ever signed up for. In the prewar era, we had been able to can or freeze food to preserve it, but now we have preservatives that can do the job—and chemicals that can boost the taste and texture lost by the manufacturing and storing processes. Why buy local raspberries in season at a farmers market when you can buy sheets of crushed and processed raspberries that are marketed as a healthy fruit substitute? Because regardless of what the sales spin is, dried raspberry "fruit leather" contains little if any fiber, more sugar than you'd eat if you were enjoying the whole fruit, and preservatives. The processed version of any food on the grocery store shelf loaded with chemicals will make you another casualty of our modern food industry.

To begin upgrading your brain, your body, and your mood, you need plant-based, nutrient-dense, and calorie-poor organic foods. By turning your kitchen into a laboratory, you can brew probiotics that can restore the health of your biome and support serotonin production and higher-brain function. You can let go of old eating habits and the sugar cravings that have been chipping away at your health, placing plants at the center of your meals and taking advantage of neuro-nutrients that enhance your brain.

To enjoy the Grow a New Brain program, you have to be willing to reduce or eliminate your intake of animal protein and dairy products for periods of time. A recent study published in *Cell Metabolism* showed that restricting the amino acid isoleucine, commonly found in eggs, dairy, and meat, increases the life span of mice by 33 percent, and reduces the incidence of cancer dramatically.[3] This would be like adding 30 more healthy years to your life! For the duration of the 10-day program in the book, you'll enjoy brain supplements and drink plant-based beverages. You will incorporate power plants into your diet, making them the centerpiece, just as your ancestors did. As a result of the lasting changes you will put into practice, you will live longer and happier.

After you upgrade serotonin production and optimize your gut flora, you will start to grow a new brain, allowing you to participate in the dreaming of a new world of health and beauty into being for yourself and your loved ones.

The Biome and Sleep

Dreaming is not just an odd or curious experience that happens at night but a hallmark of a healthy brain. Dreaming requires that we get a good night's sleep—something that, according to CDC estimates, one in three persons in the United States do not actually get.[4] To recover your ability to sleep deeply and wake up rested, you need to repair your microbiome. All roads lead back to your gut! Because you'll be supporting your microbiome with a plant-based diet, don't be surprised if you're remembering dreams again after a spell of recalling few, if any, dreams. To let you sleep through the night, the brain needs to produce melatonin. Melatonin is manufactured from serotonin by the pineal gland. In fact, it is the only hormone manufactured by this gland. That's how important it is.

Sleep repairs brain cells. Professor Lior Appelbaum, who has studied sleep with Dr. David Zada and his colleagues at Bar-Ilan University in Israel, points out, "Even jellyfish, worms, and flies sleep—but why? All animals with a nervous system sleep, but it's against evolution, against survival. If you sleep, it makes you vulnerable to predators—it doesn't make sense at all." But studies show that for humans, sleep is important for learning and memory.

That's because it enables the brain to clear out toxins and senescent cells (more on that in Chapter 9: Make Use of Powerful Pathways for Brain Health). Along with Dr. Zada, Professor Appelbaum published a study in 2019 that used zebrafish and showed that a crucial function of sleep is DNA repair. The research team observed that DNA damage in neurons increased with sleep deprivation, but other cells didn't seem to suffer. He suggests that we sleep so that our neurons can perform essential housekeeping—and that we can't do this when awake. Cumulative damage to brain cells leads to neurodegenerative disease.[5]

If you don't sleep well, preferably for at least seven hours a night, you'll end up with "brain fog" and muddled thinking. Your mood will suffer too. In short, you need your sleep, specifically, restorative, deep sleep and sleep that involves dreaming.

We know that dreams help transform short-term memories into long-term ones. And when we do not sleep deeply and restfully, this function is impaired. One of the features of AD is that long-term memories we put away into safekeeping are clear and crisp, yet short-term memories that didn't benefit from the "save" function in the brain are lost.

After my grandfather passed away, my grandmother went to live with his brother, who lived alone after having lost his wife a few years earlier. He had no short-term memory recall yet could remember in vivid detail the day of my grandmother's wedding and would remind her of how beautiful she looked as she stood at the altar. He had lost his fluid intelligence even as his crystallized intelligence remained intact. When I would visit, I would have to introduce myself. If I went to the bathroom or to the kitchen for a glass of water and returned to the room, I would have to reintroduce myself all over again, as he would exclaim, "Who are you, young man? Do I know your mother?"

This does not have to be your fate.

Key Takeaways:

We explored the realms of consciousness of the mind and how they are related to the brain.

1. How medicine men and women perform their work in the hidden realms of consciousness to interact with forces affecting the body, the brain, and the mind.

2. How the gut plays a vital role in illness and mood problems. Growing a new gut is essential for growing a new brain, influencing brain health. Friendly gut bacteria extract nutrients, support the immune system, and contribute to overall health and well-being.

Chapter 3

GROW A WISE BRAIN

Our species is called *Homo sapiens—wise human—*but given the pressures we face in our world and how clumsily we respond to them, we might have to rethink just how wise we are. Do we have the wisdom to handle our increasingly hectic lives—maintaining our presence on social media, posting new videos and messages, responding to urgent texts, staying up on our work and personal e-mail, and then giving our loved ones the attention they need from us? How will we be able to protect ourselves from deepfakes and misinformation generated by AI? Even if we are keeping up as we go forward in a time of great change that requires resilience, how long can we maintain our ability to juggle it all given the quality of brain function we have right now?

Homo sapiens evolved from an earlier protohuman whose genetic legacy can be found in every modern person. If you want to be reminded of your humble beginnings, do a mail-in genetic test and discover how much your Neanderthal cousins made a mark on your DNA. The most capable protohumans were able to thrive when environmental conditions changed and the usual food sources became scarce.

Nature is always experimenting, letting some organisms die and the most successful ones thrive. It's odd that 99 out of 100 species that once roamed the earth have perished and are now in the dust pile of prehistory. Charles Darwin considered the principle behind evolution "survival of the fittest." However, when you look at the evolution of creatures on the earth, it's brains, not brawn, that matters. The evidence of survival of the wisest is that *Homo sapiens* came to dominate over all other animals.

I first learned of this theory as a young graduate student when I had the opportunity to interview Dr. Jonas Salk for a chapter he prepared for a book I was editing (with Ken Dychtwald) called *Millennium: Glimpses into the 21st Century.* Ken and I were barely out of college and full of the chutzpah and daring of young men, and we invited 20 leading thinkers of the late 1900s, including Jonas Salk, to tell us what they thought the future might look like.

Dr. Salk is best known for developing the first effective polio vaccine. Considered one of the greatest medical achievements of the 20th century, the vaccine helped dramatically decrease the number of polio cases and ultimately led to the eradication of the polio virus in the United States. Dr. Salk made his vaccine available to all countries free of charge and received no financial benefit from his discovery.

Dr. Salk believed humanity might be following the course of lemming populations that have regular catastrophic die-offs. But while in the past the major threats to humans were from infectious diseases, today the "die-off" might already be happening due to internal challenges ranging from anxiety and stress to anger and aggression. In his chapter for our book, Dr. Salk wrote, "It is likely that the human brain has developed in the course of natural selection, partly as a result of exogenous forces active against survival. Does that same brain also possess the capacity to tame and discipline those inner forces that act against long-term survival, in opposition to a life of high-quality? The struggle for survival once manifested principally *between humanity and nature now seems to be taking place within the human species itself, between humanity and individuals*, and within individuals."[1]

In other words, the stress and trauma we're facing today no longer come from a saber-toothed tiger threatening to eat our young, but from inside our own minds. We are going mad and making each other feel that way too. We lack a sense of meaning and purpose. We don't have inner wisdom, which Dr. Salk pointed out is the most important skill we need to survive. As he explained, "We must look to those among us who are in closest touch with the unfathomable source of creativity in the human species . . ."[2] He went on to say, "Wisdom, understood as a new kind of strength, is a paramount necessity for humankind. Now, even more than ever before, it is required as a basis for fitness, to maintain life itself on the face of this planet."

When We First Had to Develop Wisdom

How did a creature that is exquisitely vulnerable at birth—with huge heads and floppy necks, unable to run from danger or do much beyond sleep, cry, eat, and poop—evolve to create philosophy, governments, music, poetry, space stations, and the World Wide Web? How did we survive plagues such as the Black Death, which wiped out at least a third of the population of Europe in the Middle Ages, and the myriad of wars we have waged against one other? As it turns out, survival of the fittest didn't mean that the fastest or fiercest creatures would come to dominate the earth. *Tyrannosaurus rex* could have ripped humans to pieces in seconds with its massive jaw and serrated teeth—but its species couldn't outcompete the swiftly moving, smaller mammals who adapted to the changing environment.

Despite our many weaknesses, early humans had something other primates lacked: a brain that could imagine, reason, and plan. We had a dawning "new brain"—the neocortex, and frontal lobes in the forehead—that gave us a huge survival advantage. The sloping brow of the Neanderthal, reminiscent of apes, gave way to foreheads and forebrains that let us outwit other species and attempt to control nature itself.

Called to Evolve Yet Again—for Good Reason

Despite our well-developed brains and the extraordinary inventions modern humans have come up with in our short 300,000 or so years on the planet, we're part of nature and must recognize her power to compel us to respond to changes in the environment. We're living on a planet that is straining under the weight of human activity. Global climate change and the massive disruptions it will cause threaten our children's future, and we need a new wisdom to innovate our way out of this dire situation.

Historically we've been on a quest to ensure that our tribe finds safety and can continue to live another day. Consequently, too many of us have forgotten our interconnectedness with one other. We've subscribed to the mindset of the conqueror—the anxiety that "it's us or them." The enemy is not "them." It is our crippling fear that we won't be safe, and that becomes a self-fulfilling prophecy when trying to procure safety by defending ourselves from our perceived enemies.

Our ancient M-brain is not only on the lookout for enemies. It *requires* enemies. Particularly the structure known as the amygdala.

The amygdala consists of two almond-shaped clusters of neurons located deep within the M-brain. It is associated with snap emotional reactions and survival instincts including fear and aggression. The amygdala is in charge of emotional decision-making in the face of threats. It needs a scapegoat to blame for the ills of the village, and that scapegoat ends up being the people with another skin color or language or religion who we are sure want our land. One appalling example of how our M-brain projects the figure of the enemy on the "other" was the Albigensian Crusade of 1209, where a Catholic abbot named Arnaud Amalric led Crusaders to sack and pillage towns in southern France, slaughtering close to one million villagers over obscure religious differences within a faith they shared. And in the last century, we have witnessed instances of mass genocide as the amygdala struggles to keep the driver's seat in our brain: the Jews in Germany, the Armenians in Turkey, the Tutsi in Rwanda, and countless more.

Fortunately, the frontal lobes of the neocortex are designed to control the amygdala and help us become more conscious of ourselves. They began waking up during the "little renaissance" in 12th-century Europe. Prior to that time, there was very little sense of individuality. Art was created "for the greater glory of

God," works were left unsigned, and craftsmen did not consider themselves separate from the collective. There was no personal fame or glory. In the year 1215, King John of England signed the Magna Carta, guaranteeing his vassals individual freedoms that would have never been possible a century before. The neocortex was reawakening after the long sleep of the Dark Ages, discovering a sense of "I" and "self."

We Can Give Up Our Species' Destructiveness

The frontal lobes of the neocortex invite us to embrace new values and see ourselves not as competitors trying to dominate each other but as peaceful collaborators. This requires quieting the amygdala, which, like a pouting, angry child wants, things its way. The frontal lobes are the adult in the room that says "take a deep breath, baby . . ."

Not all human societies have been driven into a frenzy by the amygdala. Peaceful societies have existed in Europe, Scandinavia, Malaysia, and Brazil. In fact, even today, the Cheq Wong people of Malaysia have no words to express violence, war, or even punishment.[3]

When Charles Darwin observed nature, he noticed conflict between competing species. Amazonian peoples observe nature and see a collaborative dance in which chaos and death are accompanied by creation and birth. Yes, predators kill smaller animals, but that prevents overpopulation of a species, which would disturb nature's balance. Too many of a species leads to death by starvation and disease for all. This interaction among predators and prey, among larger organisms and small microbes that can take them down as the powerful elephant dies from a bacterial infection, serves all of life.

Similarly, in our bodies, cells work together with organs and systems to create health—skin cells die every six days to be replaced by new ones. Cells that refuse to die can become tumors that spread, killing the host. Our bodies are a model of collaboration: Our cells don't compete for food or oxygen.

We have much to learn from nature's example of synergies brought about by collaboration. By working together, we don't have to overtax the earth. In all likelihood, the earth will find a way to continue despite the damage we inflict on it, but that doesn't mean we humans will be fine. If we're to live sustainably, the fear that has us on a leash to the ancient brain has to be replaced by love, awe, and humility as we step into a new way of being and learn to tread more lightly on the earth.

As an individual, you can participate, and you should, not only for the sake of the earth and others but also for your own sake.

Going from Warrior to Sage

Our nervous systems weren't designed to handle the relentless stimulation from our digital devices, which stress the amygdala in our M-brain, turning us into warriors when we need to be wise and peaceful. Twitch, the top gaming streaming site in the world, has been an active recruitment ground for the U.S. Army; the platform limits the age of players to 13 and over.[4] "Start training the future warriors young" seems to be the mandate. After all, future warfare will be digital, with pilotless planes, robots, and drones replacing the foot soldier. These video warriors live in a state of frenzy, their brains flooded with adrenaline and rewarded with dopamine, the addictive hormones that keep us under the influence of the M-brain and perceives only friend or foe and sees killing the "bad guys" as the most rewarding survival strategy.

In its crusade to remain the driver of our neural apparatus and not yield to the higher brain, the M-brain keeps us under a constant barrage of the hormone cortisol, which impairs the memory and learning center in our brain. Damage to the hippocampus leaves us no longer capable of having a new experience of life or love. We begin to age rapidly and succumb to the illnesses of aging warriors—including dementia and PTSD (even if we have never been near combat or a battlefield).

But let's take a tour through the brain's hardware, to understand what we need to upgrade to experience wisdom.

The development of the neocortex and frontal lobes was made possible by an inexplicable "accident" that occurred around some 750,000 years ago: Two chromosomes from our simian ancestors fused to form the modern human chromosome #2. (A chromosome is a DNA strand with your genetic material: 23 from your mother and 23 from your father.) This fusion resulted in our genome ending up with 46 chromosomes (while apes have 48). Chromosome #2 contains the instructions for the rapid growth of the neocortex and frontal lobes of the brain. We became the fortunate recipients of a higher and more powerful brain that allows us to use our minds to create health—or anxieties![5] We acquired the ability to turn our dreams into physical reality. We discovered how thoughts can become things.

As you kick-start your new brain, you'll break free from the addiction to adrenaline that keeps you in a battle zone, struggling with your loved ones or co-workers, producing inflammation and autoimmune disorders. (When your immune system turns against you, your body becomes the war zone. And women are most often the casualties—the collateral damage of this autoimmune conflict.) Once the pineal gland in your neocortex turns on the production of the bliss molecule DMT, you can begin to install higher-order neural networks. The brain can't produce the bliss molecule when flooded with the stress chemicals, as you cannot be preparing for peace and for war at the same time. Meanwhile, the hippocampus is rich in cortisol receptors and is damaged by cortisol. And when the hippocampus is damaged, it begins to shrink. Learning is over, school is out, and the brain prepares for war.

An Ancient Wisdom Leap

Fifty thousand years ago, as the neocortex was first coming online, humans experienced a jump in wisdom that archaeologists call "the great leap forward." Having left Africa, our ancestors migrated and settled on the banks of rivers and near large bodies of water where fish, mollusks, and mussels provided them with a food source of good fats for their brains, rich in omega-3s. These fats boost brain-derived neurotrophic factor, or BDNF, which triggers the production of stem cells in the brain. (You'll learn more about the importance of BDNF in Chapter 6: Upgrade Your Brain with BDNF.)

With abundant omega-3s, the neocortex came online in a burst of creative intensity. Humans discovered how to craft fishhooks and knitting needles and to employ bones and stones for all manner of tools. They developed art and a creativity that was previously unknown, according to archaeologists studying cave paintings our ancestors left behind in Spain and France at Altamira and Lascaux. The fish and mollusks and the primarily plant-based diet of our hunter-gatherer ancestors gave their brains the fuel and instructions needed to develop a new kind of intelligence that allowed them to survive an ice age, navigate the Pacific Ocean to settle Australia and South America, and cross the Bering Strait to North America.

We started to squander this amazing intelligence around 10,000 years ago when we domesticated corn, wheat, and rice and abandoned the omega-3-rich foods and plants we ate in our foraging days. These grains offered enough calories to stay alive. They allowed population growth—towns and cities—as grains could be stored through the winter. We began fueling our brains with carbohydrates (sugars) and stopped ingesting the nuts and plants that had kept us healthy for millennia.

It continues to this day. More than 50 percent of the food consumed in America today is ultraprocessed and loaded with sugar and bad fats. Consuming fat and sugar together triggers sensors in the stomach to signal the release of dopamine in the brain by up to 200 percent, a surge akin to the increases seen with nicotine and alcohol. And dopamine leaves us craving more. App developers know this.

The green plants in our ancestors' diets were rich in microRNAs that signaled our DNA to express the genes for health and silence the genes for disease. When we abandoned our green foraging diet, human life span declined precipitously. Instead of eating the flesh of land animals only occasionally, like we did as hunter-gatherers, we began to breed farm animals and slaughter them at our pleasure. We became voracious carnivores, and feeding on animal flesh became a sign of wealth. Not only did we lose the benefits of our previous plant-based diet, but also our diet of meat and dairy products from cows, sheep, and goats—all rich in the amino acid isoleucine—doomed our ancestors to short and brutish lives and slow and painful deaths. (Remember that restricting isoleucine, found in eggs, dairy, and meat, increases the life span of mice by 33 percent, and reduces the incidence of cancer dramatically.)

The shift to a grain-based diet was bad for individual life span but convenient for a growing population of slaves and warriors. Emperors might eat seafood regularly, but laborers would spend their days baking bricks and bread, building pyramids, and otherwise serving the higher classes with bodies fueled by grains. The Inca rulers had relay-runners known as Chaskis bring them fresh fish daily from the coast 120 miles away while their corn-fed slaves built cities in the clouds like Machu Picchu.

For the masses, the shortage of omega-3-rich foods and loss of the variety of plant foods became a sentence to inevitable senility. Their bodies no longer received instructions from the green "power plants" to switch on genes for health. Our ancestors became prone to cancers and dementia. They aged rapidly. It's as if they lost the keys to a password-protected program for health and longevity. We hear that the patriarchs in the Old Testament lived upward of 300 years. And while this may be the stuff of legend, there is no question that we are now living sicker longer than ever.

BLUE LING: FISH FOOD FOR A HEALTHY BRAIN

Garum, a fermented fish sauce, was a popular condiment in ancient Rome. And it was so highly prized that ancient Romans would pay the equivalent of $300 for a bottle of garum, a staple in their cuisine. Even the Greek poet Homer in *The Iliad* and *The Odyssey* writes about garum, whose active components appear to work synergistically to provide potent anxiolytic and antidepressant-like effects.

Excavations at Pompeii have uncovered garum production facilities, including amphorae used for storing and transporting the sauce.

While the exact date of the first use of garum in the Roman Empire is challenging to pinpoint, its presence in ancient Greek writings and its adoption by the Romans suggest that it has a long history dating back to at least the 7th century BCE.

Modern science suggests there is a reason—beyond flavor—that certain fish sauces were so prized. Garum may be a recipe for a healthy brain, as it was most likely rich in the omega-3 fatty acid DHA.

Although the lords and kings no longer live in their castles on the hills while 99 percent of the population work to support them, like they did in Medieval Europe, rampant inequality persists, and it's particularly evident in the food we eat. Most people continue to eat a paltry variety of greens—really mostly the nutrient-depleted lettuce in salads—fueling our brains on processed grains (glucose) rather than its preferred fuel of healthy fats. As a result, our brains and bodies age rapidly, and you find that the knee you twisted doesn't heal in a matter of days like it used to. Our repair systems have become sluggish, and we've lost the password to access the regeneration and longevity keys in our DNA. Our ancestors began to die young. In a paper published in 2010 in the *Proceedings of the National Academy of Sciences*, evolutionary biologist Caleb Finch describes the average life spans in ancient Greek and Roman times as approximately 20 to 35 years.[6] In contrast, our prehistoric ancestors lived to a comfortable 60 or 70 years if they survived the occasional marauding saber-toothed tigers in the first decade of life. Since 1800, human life spans have doubled again, largely due to improvements in hygiene and sanitation that greatly reduced infant mortality. Yet human health span—the number of healthy years we live—has not increased very much. We live longer sicker.

Remember, though, that doesn't have to be your destiny. We can return to the good fats like nuts, olive oil, and coconut oil—and the power plants and their microRNAs. The payoffs are enormous. You can be engaging life from your higher brain and not from the fear-based instincts of the amygdala. If you choose to participate in the experiment I am inviting you to, you can avoid losing your mind, you can snap out of the malaise and melancholy, and you can manage stressors while remaining optimistic, creative, and collaborative. You can craft a new destiny for yourself.

But first, let's look at the anatomy of the brain so you better understand the ancient regions of the brain and the recently evolved higher brain, where we can experience newfound wisdom.

Three Brains

In the mid-1950s, American neuroscientist Paul D. MacLean proposed a model to help explain the evolution of the human brain. He suggested we think of ourselves as having three evolutionarily distinct brains, each with its own intelligence, subjective sense of the world, and unique perspective. This three-brain model serves as a helpful metaphor for understanding how we react differently to experiences depending on which of the three "brains" we are primarily responding from. It explains how one person might read a situation as dangerous while another might see it as an opportunity. Consequently, there are no traumatic events, only traumatic experiences, depending on the brain you are perceiving and interpreting life from.

MacLean identified the reptilian brain (the R-brain), the mammalian brain (the M-brain), and the neocortex (the N-brain). The most primitive of these is the reptilian brain, which is anatomically much like the brain of today's reptiles. The R-brain controls our autonomic functions. It governs our breathing, our internal body temperature, our blood pressure and heart rate, our digestion, and our sexual arousal. This brain is instinctual and is interested primarily in self-preservation. There's nothing cuddly about a reptile; this brain thinks no thoughts about the meaning of life and feels no emotions. It's as cold-blooded as a snake, operating for the sole purpose of keeping you alive.

The second is the M-brain, which includes the amygdala, the hypothalamus that controls the fight-or-flight response, and the hippocampus, the learning center. It's the brain shared by all mammals and first emerged around the time that dinosaurs were facing extinction. While this brain can't reason or understand quantum physics, it's the brain of instinct and emotion. Those powers have enabled us to survive multiple ice ages. This brain believes you are at the center of the universe, and that "it's all about me." Even as Copernicus demonstrated that the Earth is not at the center of the cosmos, this brain continues to believe that you are.

The M-brain has four basic instincts, known as the Four F's—fear, feeding, fighting, and fornicating. Your M-brain may find meeting a person for the first time as an individual to be wary of or it may see a potential romantic partner. Do they present a danger or an opportunity? The M-brain is always wondering "What's in it for me?" and "What's a good strategy for keeping myself safe emotionally?" Often, its default is seeking power over others—or greed, or dishonesty, or even violence. Medieval kings were known for banishing their male offspring lest they be murdered by them, and Sigmund Freud described the Oedipus complex, the unconscious desire of the male child to slay his father and betroth his mother.

The M-brain is where you experience fear. It contains the seahorse-shaped hippocampus and the amygdalae, which are shaped like two almonds (and referred to in the singular). Your amygdala flips on the fire alarm when you perceive a threat. The fight-or-flight system springs into action. Think about the last time you felt frightened. Your heart raced and you felt a burst of energy rushing through you because of the cortisol and adrenaline pumping though your system. Your instinct was to flee as quickly as possible or put up the fight of your life. Maybe you froze, completely shut down in a primitive response that turned you into the opossum playing dead.

The fight-or-flight response can snap on even when a threat isn't an actual danger but merely a perceived one. Have you ever read a news report that made you so angry that you felt the changes in your body and the response that I described? If so, it's because your M-brain needs a reset. Even when you're not aware, it is creating dark moods, making you certain our world is going to pot, like your life is a fierce fight for survival, and turning you into an armchair warrior, scanning for threats to your well-being.

If you have ever been in danger, I'm sure you appreciated your reptilian and M-brains. If you fell on a hike far from any medical help and had a cut or bleeding limb, you wouldn't have to tell your body what to do: It knows how to respond. As adults, we tend to take for granted our body's ability to heal itself. The reptilian and M-brains served us well during the millennia we lived in the wilds, but it is not the part of your brain where you can experience joy, curiosity, or bliss. Let's not forget the importance of the third, higher brain—the neocortex or N-brain, which contains the frontal lobes some scientist are calling the "God Spot."

More recently evolved, the neocortex (neo means "new" and cortex means "outer") is the outside layer of your brain—the gray matter—that is wrinkled like a walnut so that more surface area can fit inside your cranium, allowing you plenty of territory for processing original thoughts. Unlike even our closest simian relatives, the chimpanzees, we have well-developed frontal lobes, which we use when planning, imagining, and daydreaming. The N-brain is the brain of poets, scientists, and philosophers, and it's where we experience selfless love, compassion, reasoning, and logic. Using this higher brain, we can craft musical compositions, create works of art, discover new technologies, entertain ideas such as democracy and quantum physics, and envision the future we want for ourselves and our loved ones. This is the brain of spirituality, not of religion, which thrives with the M-brain.

This N-brain developed because of that uncanny fusion of chromosome #2 millennia ago and first came online some 50,000 years ago when we took a leap in our wisdom to discover art and new technologies. This is the brain we want guiding our moods, thoughts, perceptions, and actions, even as our more primitive brains look after our well-being. Yet most of humanity is still sputtering along on the stale-dated M-brain that perceives our neighbor as our enemy and fights and bickers over whose god is more powerful. We need the higher brain if we're to evolve and see the world not as a dangerous place filled with enemies but as an enchanted creation that we contribute to and that supports us—as long as we have a reciprocal and sustainable relationship with it. Much as we don't like to admit it, we tend to treat the earth like we treat our own mothers, taking her for granted and assuming she will always be there to take care of us, while still blaming her for all *our* shortcomings. The N-brain is realizing that Mom's exhausted, that we must stop straining her resources and taxing her ability to support life.

In addition, we have the frontal lobes, part of our N-brain, in our foreheads. It's the brain that views with the eyes of the eagle, which flies high above, taking in a broad perspective of the land, its rivers and trees, and even the mouse scurrying into the bushes. In the Amazon, the sages speak of seeing beyond the limits of our everyday perception. With eagle perception, we experience the wisdom that allows us to master epigenetics, using our thoughts to turn on genes for health and turning off genes for disease—a form of wisdom we have available to us but that far too few know how to use. But this is just the beginning. The wisdom this new brain offers will not only allow you to break free from your genetic fate and create psychosomatic wellness, but it will also allow you to use your eagle vision to craft a meaningful destiny. It will enable you to understand the laws of the universe—the implicate order—and learn to interact creatively with them for dreaming your world and your health into being.

Our frontal lobes enabled our ancestors to thrive after the last glacial period. When the ice began to recede, they were able to migrate to the lush valleys following the game and the nuts and berries. Our distant relatives, the Neanderthals, lacked frontal lobes. They had to rely on routines ingrained in ritual and religion, such as the habit of not going farther than a half day's trek away from the home cave, which caused them to miss out on the opportunities presented by a more favorable climate in the lush valleys. The N-brain allowed humans to understand the cycles of nature, fertility, the movement of the stars, and animal migration. And while the M-brain could lead you back to the tree with the great walnuts, it would not be able to help you anticipate the movement of the buffalo herds.

Our ancient M-brain holds on to outdated maps and beliefs and behaviors. No matter how much evidence you present to its owner, you won't be able to convince their M-brain that the world is round or that we have sent astronauts to the moon. This brain will choose to feel miserable rather than to lose an argument.

While the R-brain changes through the promise of food or the threat of pain, the M-brain needs ceremonies if it is to change. It will not change when presented with facts. This is why every culture around the world has ceremonies and rites of passage that mark transitions where you go from an old way to a new way or role, accompanied by a change in status in the community—for example puberty, menopause, marriage, manhood and womanhood, including college graduation and weddings.

FIRE CEREMONY FOR TRANSFORMATION

Because we spent a million years sitting around the fire, it's almost in our DNA to gather around the campfire and share its warmth and sense of safety. Many Indigenous traditions use fire or smoke from burning sage or other sweet herbs (or incense) during ceremonies. They understood that to achieve genuine change, we need ceremony. Otherwise, the M-brain will keep us stuck in the known, clinging to the familiar.

You cannot change your mind unless you change your brain. The higher brain changes through bliss, through an experience of Oneness, of communion, with the help of serotonin and DMT, but the lower M-brain needs ceremony. These are found in every culture, from wedding ceremonies to birth and death rites to rituals marking the passage into adulthood. If we miss out on these rites, we don't grow. You can create your own ceremonies as long as they are infused with meaning for you!

The fire ceremony can serve to transform a memory of trauma that has never truly healed. Remember: Traumas from childhood can linger in your body and continue to influence your emotions. You can use this ceremony to transform trauma into wisdom.

Trauma is the way we remember what occurred to us. We wrap a story around it, which can make it extremely difficult for us to interpret our past experience in a different way. The fire ceremony will allow you to "offer" the story and the emotions associated with it into a stick called a "death arrow" that you will place in the fire, freeing yourself from the tale and bringing its healing energy into your heart to recover its power.

Free yourself from the tyranny of a story about what caused a wound in you (and maybe in another person too). You'll be using your breath to blow the emotions and people involved into this "death arrow," so that the fire can transform your trauma and release how the story lives within you. Remember, there are no traumatic events, only traumatic experiences!

To conduct your fire ceremony, first identify a painful experience you would like to transform. Then, get a candle (such as a tealight) and a small stick (such as a toothpick) that you can burn in the flame.

Set your intention for releasing the story that has held you in its grip for a long time. Then, light the candle. Next, hold the toothpick to your lips and blow into it the memory of your experience—the emotions in your heart. Blow into the stick your feelings for the people who hurt you, who didn't help or rescue you. Blow into it the names of the people involved, and if you can, forgive them for the lessons that they offered you despite the terrible way you suffered as a result.

Hold this stick to the fire. Watch it burn. When the stick is extinguished safely, pass your hands over the flame, drawing the fire's warmth toward your heart. Bring this energy, this light, into your heart center as the old story fades and is replaced by the lessons that life has offered you.

Once you have transformed a memory, you will start to discover that you are not the story anymore. You are becoming the storyteller of your own life.

And you will craft stories that support your wisdom and success.

Many people are convinced that the story of Genesis is the literal truth about how the earth came into being. Yet with time, science began to erode the power of the priests, with an alternative explanation of the origins of life. The N-brain provided us with a better explanation than the one provided by religion as to who we are and our origins. Now we can use the same neural resources to discover who we are at the core when we're not driven by fear, scarcity, or violence against ourselves and others. But if we operate from the lower M-brain, there will be no creativity, generosity, or evolution in consciousness. That's because this brain can flip the switch to the fire alarm on a moment's notice and the amygdala will hijack the higher brain and start looking for someone to blame.

The Hypothalamus, the Amygdala, and Danger!

The hypothalamus is the command center for the release of hormones by the pituitary. When you are attracted to another person, the hypothalamus releases oxytocin, one of the "happy hormones," so you can bond and "fall in love." Your hypothalamus also manages many "body harmonizing" functions by influencing the nervous system, which has two components: the sympathetic and the parasympathetic nervous system. The sympathetic nervous system is like the gas pedal in a car, turning on "do or die," while the parasympathetic nervous system is like the brake, sending you into a "rest and digest" response.

The hypothalamus is like a thermostat that can be adjusted. This is called the set point. It determines at what level of perceived danger you begin to get alarmed. Early life trauma influences our hypothalamus's set point, determining when it sends a signal up to the higher brain (OPPORTUNITY) or down to the amygdala (DANGER). People who have experienced childhood trauma have brains that are more fragile, making it harder for them to regulate their chemical and emotional response to a perceived danger.[7] Researcher Seymour Levine studied rats and found that in those who experienced maternal affection as infants, "their cortisol secretion was diminished, and this reduction persisted into adulthood."[8] These animals had a higher hypothalamus set point, so it took a greater sense of danger to flag their M-brain to release cortisol and go into hyperdrive.

Normal cortisol levels peak early in the morning to help you bound out of bed and greet the day. Chronically high *or* low levels make you feel fatigued and exhausted. We want our cortisol level fluid and the set point of the hypothalamus to be such that we aren't sensing danger everywhere. But remember, this setting was programmed by how safe you felt during your life in-utero and your childhood. While we can't change our past, we can change both how it affects us and our hypothalamus's set point. We don't want to disable the "thermostat" of the fight-or-flight system. We just want to ensure that it alerts us to *real* danger, not imaginary ones.

We want to be able to see opportunities that we would otherwise miss, and respond with openness and curiosity.

Early in my career as an anthropologist, I spent many months in the jungle in Peru studying the medicine plants. At that time, the country was overrun by Maoist guerrillas. There was a constant danger of being robbed of all your belongings (including your vital organs!) in the Wild West jungle ports from which I launched my expeditions. As a result, I always carried my passport in a money belt inside my pants and kept a tight hold on my camera (and my kidneys). I was never robbed in the Amazon, but the fear stayed with me. When my research project ended, I returned to New York to brief the organization that sponsored me. The directors took me to a nice restaurant for lunch and mentioned to me that I was holding tight to my camera even while eating. I realized I was still carrying my money in my belt and scanning the restaurant for potential danger! I reminded myself that I was back in the United States and could relax again. But I had not changed the set point of my hypothalamus, so I was still looking for threats from the waiters! Even today, I occasionally catch myself scanning a restaurant or train station for danger and have to breathe deeply—I like using the 4:4 breath here—to lower the set point of my fight-or-flight system.

THE 4:4 BREATHING PRACTICE

The "4-4-4" breathing practice is a simple and effective way to soothe the mind and brain. It consists of a cycle of deeply inhaling for four counts, pausing and holding the breath for four counts, followed by a gradual exhale over four counts, and holding the breath empty for four counts. This practice helps diminish anxiety while inducing relaxation. To practice this technique, find a peaceful and comfortable space where you can sit or recline. Begin by inhaling deeply through your nose, ensuring your lungs are full, and exhale deeply. Repeat and exhale.

Next, inhale to a count of four, hold your breath for four counts, gradually exhale through your nose for four counts, making sure all air is expelled from your lungs, and hold empty for four counts. Continue this breathing pattern for a few minutes until you achieve a state of relaxation. This is a great aid for falling asleep at night!

Keeping our hypothalamus at a reasonable set point makes life less scary, and we are less likely to respond to threats that aren't real, so it doesn't damage our brain. The hypothalamus is responsible for the amount of cortisol our adrenal glands release, signaling to them to keep pumping it out, even when this means dooming the hippocampus to destruction—because cortisol damages that vital structure of the brain.

What's more, if you're not upgrading your hypothalamus, you become prone to obesity and diabetes. That's because cells called tanycytes are responsible for neurogenesis in the hypothalamus of adults. Tanycytes help control body weight and energy balance to prevent putting on excess pounds. If you are not able to shed the weight, it could be due to your hypothalamus needing repair.

Fortunately, as Swedish neurologist Peter Eriksson discovered, we all have stem cells that can become brain neurons.[9] The Grow a New Brain program will help you tap into this wealth of cells, from which all brain cells are made.

The Wisdom We Need

Knowledge can help you memorize information to ace a multiple-choice test—and now that we have AI, having facts is less valuable than ever. Machines can take care of the facts now better than we can, as we have outsourced many of our brain's memory functions to our digital devices. But wisdom is much harder to attain than rote knowledge. Having the definition of a word, or whether something can be categorized as this or that, is different from having good judgment in making decisions on how to best use our gifts and skills. To discover a new way of wisdom, we need to grow the *gifts* of our N-brain.

One of the most valuable is holistic wisdom. In the West, our approach to life is not holistic. We don't consider mental, emotional, physical, and spiritual health to be related. We wait for something to go wrong with our body and then attack it with an "anti"—an anti-inflammatory, an antibiotic, an antidepressant, etc. Our thinking is reductionist. We see the body as a collection of parts. The GI specialists deal with our digestion and the psychiatrists and psychologists work with the mind and the brain, not realizing that much of what goes wrong in the mind comes from the gut. The neurologists claim the brain as theirs and the cardiologists the heart, forgetting that the heart has a brain of its own with more than 40,000 neurons.

The French anthropologist Claude Lévi-Strauss once commented that before we Westerners could understand the workings of the cosmos we had to understand the working of a blade of grass. Modern scientists can explain how grass turns sunlight into life through the process of photosynthesis. But for the Indigenous sage, before you can understand the workings of a blade of grass, you have to discern the workings of the cosmos. The higher brain can achieve this holistic perspective through intuitive insight, or gnosis. Like Henry David Thoreau said, "It's not what you look at that matters, it's what you see."

We have lost sight of the horizon and no longer see the curvature of the earth. The M-brain can help us spot dangers, but the N-brain lets us discover opportunities. The higher brain enables us to sense the unlimited possibilities available to us when we experience the wisdom of the living cosmos. I felt this many times in the Amazon during ceremonies with the plant medicine. I was able to converse with the rainforest—and she answered every question I had even before I had a chance to formulate them. I was shown that there is an underlying reality that can only be understood through experience. The sages call it that which "can be known but not told."

As the poet Johann Wolfgang von Goethe said, "Assuredly, there is no more lovely worship of God than that for which no image is required, but which springs up in our breast spontaneously when nature speaks to the soul, and the soul speaks to nature face to face."

Upgrading Our Hardware

Who wouldn't want to develop the superpower to turn off the genes for illness and disease and turn on the genes for health and longevity? We acquire this power with the help of the plants. They hold the secret for controlling gene expression to override the aging and senescence we seem to be destined for.

Until we upgrade the brain with the power plants, and provide it with the precursors for serotonin, we'll continue on the same path to unnecessary frailty, suffering, and diseases of aging, which can start in your early 30s. In a sense, we need to return to the garden—the paradise that we've been told we were kicked out of—to rediscover our relationship with the plants. Ask a villager in the Amazon, "How do you know which shrub to brew into a calming tea?" and you will get the answer, "The plants speak to me."

When I first heard this, I didn't know what to make of that answer. Over time, I came to realize that much as I value the scientific method of discovery, we shouldn't undervalue the Indigenous wisdom ways. How powerful are they? If you were to prepare curare, a neurotoxin used on the tips of hunters' arrows, which became the basis of anesthesia in the West, you would have to follow strict instructions. You would take deadly moonseed flowers and the bark of *Strychnos toxifera* and slowly cook them for hours until the brew becomes a dark, syrupy paste. If you were to accidentally inhale its sweet vapors, your chest muscles would stop working, you would go into convulsions and not be able to call for help—and soon, you would asphyxiate. Those who prepare it watch it brew from a safe distance, knowing the danger of inhaling its fumes—or touching it if they have a cut that's a doorway into their bloodstream. Had the first hunters used trial and error to perfect their recipe, many would have died in the discovery process.

The hunters I met in an Amazonian village renowned for its curare told me that the reason they knew how to make this deadly toxin was because "the plants explained it to us." Later that day, I decided to ask a very big, wise-looking chiwawako (iron tree) if it would show me the plants that cure AD, but I got no response. When I shared this with my hunter friend, he explained, "It didn't know what to say. We don't have this 'Alzheimer's' you speak of."

Perhaps I was asking the wrong questions. If New York is not in your map, nobody can tell you how to get there.

But what I'm describing—listening to the plants—can be thought of as the active dialogue with nature. And it's one that we can reestablish. The N-brain understands that through intuitive insight, we can converse with the rivers and the trees and Spirit as Indigenous peoples do. The 10-day Grow a New Brain program will help you make your way back to the garden and discover the wisdom in the sacred plants there, and perhaps find their voice again.

Here's another example of ancient wisdom that predated modern science. University of Adelaide microbiologist Laura Weyrich studied the plaque in the teeth of Neanderthal jaw bones found at El Sidrón, Spain, and found evidence that our extinct cousins consumed poplar bark, known to be rich in salicylic acid, the active ingredient in aspirin, making it effective for pain relief from a toothache.[10] Europeans would not discover the secret the Neanderthals were onto until 1897, when German chemist Felix Hoffmann invented aspirin by processing salicylic acid into acetylsalicylic acid.[11] Dr. Hoffmann would later go on to found the largest pharmaceutical conglomerate in the world, F. Hoffmann-La Roche & Co. (today, Roche Pharmaceuticals).

Our Capacity to Help Ourselves

Too often, we look to others to rescue us—and blame them when they can't or won't do that. Look at our relationship with physicians. Traditionally, we have exalted them, as if they have magical powers we lack, but what physicians really do is help us help ourselves. It's our bodies that do the healing; the treatments simply facilitate (or hinder) the work. We can always choose to partner with skilled doctors, but their job is to help the body repair itself, not to "fix" us.

We can engage the higher brain's capacity to protect our health by learning to activate the placebo mechanism. This effect, well known among medical researchers, refers to our strange ability to respond to a pill with inert ingredients (sugar, fillers, etc.) as if it were an effective medication. A sugar pill can reduce pain as much as morphine can in 56 percent of people.[12] It does so not by fooling the body but by turning on the brain's pharmaceutical factories to produce the chemicals that reduce pain and inflammation. And curiously, the mechanism works even when a patient knows that they are receiving a placebo! The mind's ability to cue the body to heal and repair itself may be mysterious—we don't know its mechanisms—but it's undeniably powerful and available to us.

As a young researcher, working in a lab surrounded by the pickled brains of strangers, I tried to find how the brain can create psychosomatic health. What I learned from the Amazon sages I met was that instead of focusing on the brain, I should have been also focusing on the mind. I underestimated the mind's ability to create health (and illness too). When the mind aligns with the living grid of wisdom we are part of, the potential for healing increases exponentially. Miracles happen.

Just as real as the placebo effect is that of its opposite, the nocebo effect, where the mind creates illness by the power of belief. Years ago, I was working near the headwaters of the Marañón River, in Peru, when I met a man who said he'd been "cursed" by a neighbor. The man came to a village elder for help with the head-splitting migraines he had been experiencing. The elder said there was nothing to do to help him. In fact, he told the man to go home to his family and break the bad news so they would be prepared for him to die.

I was quite surprised by the pronouncement, as the man seemed perfectly healthy. How could he know from his simple observation that the man was doomed? I said nothing, but the next week, I learned that the man had become sick. A month later he died.

I was shocked, and my inquisitive mind sought answers. I went to the same elder that the man had seen the month before and, trying to keep the irritation out of my voice, I asked, "Why didn't you help him?" The healer explained that the man had broken a village taboo, a serious one that would affect many others. It was his own guilt that had killed him.

I was confused. "Do you mean the curse was only in his mind?"

"No," the healer said. "I know the sorcerer who cursed him. He is very powerful."

Back then I did not believe in sorcerers and curses. But like the distressed man who came for healing, we have minds that can persuade our bodies to manifest illness or miraculous cures. Our fears can get the better of us and hijack our emotions, such as when we get a terrible medical diagnosis and find ourselves in panic—a kind of modern curse. Yet spontaneous healing is more common than we think. In a carefully designed study, researchers found that 22 percent of breast cancer cases underwent spontaneous regression without treatment.[13] The authors concluded: "It appears that some breast cancers detected by repeated mammographic screening would not persist to be detectable by a single mammogram at the end of 6 years." Science can't explain why this happens. We can't either, but we have the capacity to do it.

We are starting to recognize the power of the N-brain to make us well, and direct the body to do the same, quieting the production of the stress hormones and manufacturing the bliss hormones that can create psychosomatic health.

You might not recognize the power of the stress hormones—adrenaline and cortisol—on your brain, your thoughts, and your moods. On the plus side, you may have heard of amazing feats of strength (called hysterical strength) powered by adrenaline. Think of a mother lifting a car to free her child, pinned under the vehicle, or fighting a wandering bear threatening to attack her family. But when the bears you are running into are emotional or your abusive spouse or co-workers, the stress hormones are freakishly destructive to the brain. Many of us are good at compartmentalizing our feelings during stressful situations but collapse in exhaustion or get sick after pushing through our challenges. This is perhaps the most destructive exercise we can put the hippocampus through.

When we quiet the stress hormones and find peace within our brain, the mind and the world can follow. The N-brain understands we are creating our experience of the world, but the M-brain doesn't always feel that way. More often, we feel we're the victims of a reality someone else thought up and imposed on us. The resourcefulness of our higher brain can help us live not as if life is a problem to be solved but a treasure chest to be explored.

When we create potent higher-order neural networks, we can begin to see the world with enthusiasm and understand our place in the cosmos. But to do this, we need the help of stem cells. The biggest bank of stem cells in the brain is in the hippocampus. But when the hippocampus is damaged by prolonged cortisol exposure, we lose viable stem cells. They become worn-out and exhausted and unable to repair the brain. In later chapters, you'll discover how serotonin repairs the hippocampus, and how to increase stem cell production with BDNF (brain-derived neurotrophic factors) induced by the omega-3 fatty acid DHA.

Until we upgrade our brain, we're not going to be able to change the life trajectory selected by our emotional wounds and encoded in networks in our M-brain. Our perspective will be dominated by tunnel vision, seeing only the tree and missing the forest. Fortunately, we can change our minds more easily once we upgrade our brains and are able to approach life with originality and optimism. Next, you'll learn more about how to achieve that goal.

Key Takeaways:

We explored historical and evolutionary themes related to stress.

1. The impact of human activity on the planet and the need for new wisdom to address global crises.

2. The historical development of human thinking from a tribal, survival-focused perspective to a more interconnected and planetary-focused one.

3. The impact of stress and anxiety on the brain, and techniques for managing stress, including the 4:4 breathing practice.

4. The importance of maintaining a healthy fight-or-flight set point in the hypothalamus to reduce fear and prevent damage to the hippocampus, while addressing potential health issues like obesity and diabetes.

5. The distinction between knowledge and wisdom, and the significance of wisdom in making wise decisions and utilizing skills creatively.

Chapter 4

THE PROMISE
OF THE
HIGHER BRAIN

*A great many people think they are thinking when they
are merely rearranging their prejudices.*

— DAVID BOHM

"It's impossible," I insisted to my guide. I had already shared with him my list of reasons for why we wouldn't be able to reach the remote Andean village by nightfall.

"You have found all the reasons why we can't, and none of the reasons we can," my friend said as he stood beside me under a rapidly setting sun.

"But we've run out of options."

Don Antonio shrugged. "You think I am asking you to change the sun and moon and stars. I am only asking you to change your mind so that we will arrive in the village on time."

As a Westerner, I had to become used to the Andean people's relationship to time, which was quite different from the one I had. My sense of time required the use of a clock and involved ideas like "late" and "early." I wanted to make the best use of my time here in the mountains and not waste it on conversations about how we were going to get to our destination before the thick night enveloped us in black.

I had been taught to focus on problems that needed solving, not wasting a moment in my quest to achieve my goals. Now, while I stood alongside the river with Don Antonio, the sun's rays were waning. I didn't have a vehicle or even a burro and didn't know how my guide and I could walk any faster. My hiking boots were making my feet sweat, and I wasn't sure I would be warm enough in my clothes overnight. I hadn't packed properly. I hadn't planned well enough.

Observing how anxious I looked, the old man said, "You think options all come from here" as he pointed to my head. "My ideas come from here." As he spoke, he swept an outstretched arm and hand across the landscape. Then he returned his gaze to me. "You are trapped, and you built the cage you live in."

Did we get to the village that night? No. But we did encounter locals who offered to let us stay with them in their stone hut. *Lucky coincidence*, I thought. But as I laid my head down on the folded blanket they had offered me and settled myself to go to sleep, the maestro spoke through the darkness.

"You think we're here by luck, but we are not. We are here because I am part of a greater destiny. I spoke to Pachamama, I asked her to help us reach the village on time, and she told me to keep walking along the riverbank, to take our time."

"Mmm," I replied. I was irritated with Don Antonio for telling me again about being in the flow with nature, but was too tired to argue.

The next day, Don Antonio insisted we stay for a while, as our host had prepared a rich breakfast of homegrown purple potatoes. It was not until the day after that we finally set off to our destination. We arrived as night was falling, and a young man hurried to meet us.

"Ah! You're here! We had intense rain the night before that turned the footpath to mud. The trail was nearly washed away completely. It's fortunate you didn't come earlier."

The old man glanced over at me, and I could swear that inside, he was laughing. We had arrived in perfect time.

Solutions Come from a New Map

The brain switches to autopilot whenever possible, freeing our frontal lobes to imagine and daydream as our lower brains guide us on familiar paths. This ability is helpful if we have to get to work on time and travel along the usual route. Our brain's map for getting us out the door and to our workplace is not so helpful if we are driving elsewhere—to an appointment or to go grocery shopping because it's our day off. We'll find ourselves on the usual road thinking, "Idiot me! I forgot to take the exit! I'm so used to driving to work . . ."

Now more than ever, we can't be on autopilot. We can't behave the way we always have, relying on our usual knowledge base by only engaging the things that are already familiar to us. Autopilot isn't serving us—and neither is the habit of thinking that if we can't figure out how to craft a new destination for ourselves, it's okay to let ourselves become irritated and demand that someone fix it for us.

We've become used to spinning a story about who did what to whom. Someone's the bad guy (not us!), someone's the victim, and someone's the noble rescuer. Maybe we're the noble rescuer of the victim, which justifies our harsh judgment of the person we perceive as the aggressor. We can't possibly be the jerk in the scenario. The tales we tell ourselves keep us in unproductive, painful dramas. And they are tales spun by our ancient M-brain and the three major actors it has in its repertoire: victim, perpetrator, and rescuer—ancient characters in a modern drama that keeps us from achieving what we want and leaves us with the reasons why we can't.

While few of us would admit that we think this way, remember back to the last time you had a problem with travel arrangements that was going to cost you time and money, or maybe you just found yourself in the wrong line after waiting there for 20 minutes. My guess is that irritability shut off your creative juices and made you want to vent to someone who would solve your dilemma and soothe your emotions with a flurry of apologies. You probably wondered, "Where is that intelligent and sensitive person who will save me from the idiot that's screwing up my reservation?" Too often, the world seems to be conspiring to ruin our day for us.

Remember our M-brain has only these three roles in its repertoire when things go wrong. Allowing our M-brain to send us into a fearful, angry response, we fight the flow of life and inhibit our ability to co-create a harmonious reality. You might not know how to solve a particular problem, but fresh ideas can come to you when you're in a higher state of consciousness. What if the solution is something you have yet to imagine? Imagination requires an entirely different set of hormones and neural networks than those that support the roles of victim, perpetrator, and rescuer.

When we allow ourselves to dream a bigger dream than merely managing life well enough to not suffer unnecessarily, we step off the habitual paths etched into the M-brain networks. Neural networks are information superhighways formed by brain cells that fire together and later, wire together. This is known as Hebb's law, after Donald Hebb, who explained how the brain learns and stores new information: When two neurons fire at the same time, the links between them strengthen. This process, known as synaptic plasticity (because the connections are formed between the neurons' synapses), plays a crucial role in learning new skills. In essence, neural networks are paths we take again and again to reach the same destinations and conclusions. They serve as paths in maps—trails created by your upbringing, and particularly childhood trauma, and reside in your M-brain.

Past traumas shape our brain more than we realize—and these events aren't limited to the ones you experienced personally. In the Amazon they call them generational curses.

A study at Emory University found that the grandchildren of mice who had been shocked while exposed to a cherry blossom experienced a fear of that scent even when they were not raised near their traumatized grandparent.[1] And it's not just mice that pass on trauma generationally. An Icahn School of Medicine at Mount Sinai research team lead by Rachel Yehuda, Ph.D., discovered that children of Holocaust survivors were more likely to have an epigenetic marker related to PTSD and depression than children of Jewish descent whose parents did not live through the Holocaust in Europe.[2]

Native American sages believe that your actions will have an impact for seven generations. Today we are discovering the mechanisms that support this, how our grandmothers "live within us" so to speak.

In another study, Yehuda and her colleagues examined 187 pregnant women who had survived the collapse of the World Trade Center on September 11, 2001. Then, nine months after the initial visit, 38 women returned to Mount Sinai Hospital with their newborn children for further testing. Dr. Yehuda discovered that many of these mothers had PTSD, yet despite the stress they had undergone, the mothers had unusually low levels of the stress hormone cortisol.[3] It turns out that even though cortisol is released when you're under stress, it also inhibits the production of adrenaline and of itself in the long term.

Dr. Yehuda's discovery turns on its head the long-accepted thesis that stress results in long-term high levels of cortisol. Thanks to her research, we now know that low levels of cortisol reliably indicate long-term and intergenerational trauma. Dr. Yehuda concludes: "Epigenetics potentially explains why effects of trauma may endure long after the immediate threat is gone, and it is also implicated in the diverse pathways by which trauma is transmitted to future generations."[4]

Do you find yourself chronically fatigued? Do you have poor appetite? Is it hard to get out of bed in the morning? All of these are symptoms of low cortisol levels, and possible intergenerational trauma. Even if we think we don't bear the scars of our ancestors' pain, we are all the children and grandchildren of war and high-stress experiences—think of the Great Depression of 100 years ago—that wired our grandparents for scarcity, etching indelible neural networks in their M-brain. And we inherited these, some of us perhaps are driven to become overachievers. Remember that the stress hormones go right through the placental barrier and create toxic neural pathways (and their beliefs) in our brain when we are still in our mother's womb.

You don't have to be held hostage by a fearful brain. An upgraded brain will allow you to think clearly, free of the fog so many of us live with, but it can do much more as well. It can recognize possibilities that are hidden from you when you're acting from painful memories and emotions buried in your M-brain that lead you to believe you are in the wrong place at the wrong time with the wrong people around you.

In contrast, the higher brain understands that you are exactly where you need to be and that there are gifts even in the most challenging times. The neocortex allows you to smile at the attendant at the check-in counter at the airport instead of snarling at him. When you do that, it increases the chances that you'll get lucky and be upgraded for no reason at all. When the doctor says to you, "I have bad news," you want the higher brain's perspective, not the M-brain's panic. The N-brain understands that whatever happens must be a gift; otherwise, it wouldn't be happening. And you will begin to think, "Why is this happening *for* me?" instead of "Why is this happening *to* me?" Your gratitude will be strong no matter what is taking place in your life. And then you will realize that you have the power to select your destiny in the face of any odds, because you have a blissful dialogue with nature and the underlying fabric of creation.

David Bohm, one of the most important physicists of the 20th century, who made groundbreaking contributions to quantum theory and neuropsychology, suggested there is an "implicate order" that underlies all that we can observe and that we call reality. He is commonly attributed as saying, "Space is not empty. It is full, a plenum as opposed to a vacuum, and is the ground for the existence of everything, including ourselves. The universe is not separate from this cosmic sea of energy."

Bohm considered that ordinary reality—all beings and things, including the clouds and canyons and you and I—are only a superficial expression that emerges out of an underlying implicate order from which everything is born. The higher brain, which recognizes that we are all interconnected, you, me, the forests and the eagles and the stars, allows us to co-create with this implicate order versus only moving the furniture around in the explicate outer order.

This implicate order has been called by many names: The Andean shamans call her Pachamama or Mother Earth; the Tibetans call her Mother of the Buddhas; my friend the physicist Ervin Laszlo calls it the Akashic Field, diverse scientists call it the Quantum Field, while native peoples use the term Spirit.

Carl Jung called it the collective unconscious that speaks to us through dreams, and occasionally, through synchronicities that punctuate our lives, from small ones like seeing triple digits on a clock when you pick up your mobile phone, to amazingly uncanny meetings and opportunities that we attribute to serendipity. As I was writing these lines, I tapped my phone and it showed me the time was 12:12, confirming this!

Indigenous sages know that serendipitous events offer the possibility for co-creating a new destiny for yourself and your village. It's called "dreaming your world into being." When we do not dream our world, we have to settle for the nightmare being dreamed by the collective mass of humanity. We call it statistics and probability. The danger is that we can easily become a medical statistic that can be difficult to recover from.

This is not pretty. Statistics predict our health to be in the big fat part of the bell curve, where we will age and get sick and die like most Americans. And it makes us feel utterly alone and disconnected from the fabric of the implicate order.

Dream of a New Dream

While we may not find ourselves thinking often about old traumas, they continue to affect our biology until we recognize our fears and dismantle their outdated beliefs. Many of us share a belief that the way to a better life is to work ourselves to death to achieve financial security so we can enjoy our later years. In quiet moments, we wistfully long for a new way of living, but have no clue how to change the chronic stress we live under.

A 2009 study from Portugal showed that mice subjected to chronic stress lose their ability to break repetitive behavior patterns.[5] They forget how to be creative, so solutions to their problems escape them. Stress researcher and neurobiologist from Stanford University School of Medicine Robert Sapolsky said about this study, "This is a great model for understanding why we end up in a rut, and then dig ourselves deeper and deeper into that rut . . . we're lousy at recognizing when our normal coping mechanisms aren't working."[6]

Remember, it isn't brawn that will help us survive and evolve as our environment changes; it's wisdom. It's not exactly wise to keep doing the same thing repeatedly and expect different results. That's the definition of insanity.

Once the N-brain recognizes that the coping methods we've relied on in the past are dysfunctional it will start shifting us into a mindset where we replace fear with love and courage.

From Survival to Omniscience

When your M-brain is in charge, you maintain an instinctual, primitive focus on survival and selfish behavior. "What's in it for me" is your mantra. This can serve you in the short term during a crisis where you have to fight, to stand up for yourself and speak the truth or cower in fear, remaining silent. But being obsessed with fighting, fleeing, feeding, and sexually manipulating other people isn't conducive to healthy long-term relationships. You become trapped in the nightmare we call human history. When you are thinking with your M-brain, you're perceiving more than what is true at a literal level. You can sense that night is falling—you are right about that. You can observe it with your eyes. But you perceive something else too: danger. It's all around you, in the darkness, in the unknown.

What we need is to quiet our M-brain and not let it run away in fear and miss a great opportunity. Let me illustrate how the M-brain can miss the best possibility when it only thinks selfishly about its own survival. The prisoner's dilemma is a problem in the field of game theory. It presents a scenario where two individuals, acting selfishly, might not cooperate, even though it would be in their best interest to do so.

Imagine two criminals, A and B, are arrested and imprisoned. Each prisoner is in solitary confinement with no means of communicating with the other. The prosecutors lack sufficient evidence to convict the pair on the principal charge, but they have enough to convict both on a lesser charge. The prosecutors offer each prisoner a bargain:

1. If A and B both confess to the major crime (betray each other), each will serve two years in prison.

2. If A confesses but B denies the crime, A will be freed (as an incentive for confessing), and B will serve three years in prison (for the major crime), and vice versa.

3. If both A and B deny the crime (cooperate with each other), both will serve only one year in prison (for the lesser charge).

The dilemma arises because each prisoner has a choice between two options, neither of which depends on the other: to cooperate with their fellow prisoner by remaining silent, or to betray the other by confessing. The best outcome for both prisoners is if they both cooperate and serve only one year. However, without being able to trust the other person to remain silent, each prisoner individually faces the temptation to confess and possibly go free at the expense of the other serving three years.

The prisoner's dilemma shows why two completely rational individuals might not cooperate, even if it appears that it is in their best interests to do so.

How would you choose to respond?

Jaguar Medicine

In the Amazon, the jaguar represents the power and fearless instinct we awaken when we overcome fear by acknowledging it and transforming it into courage. Just as courage is the absence of fear, the reverse is also true. Fear is the absence of courage. When we embody the energy and qualities of the jaguar, who has no predators, our fear starts to fade as we choose courage and curiosity and learn that the universe is benign and supporting us *always*.

For a long time, psychologists told us that if we would just face our fear and learn from it, we could rise above it. But that's only true if you have a brain with an undamaged hippocampus, which is where our "maps" of reality are crafted. As you upgrade the hippocampus you realize you are only afraid of the dark because of what you *believe* lies lurking in the shadows. You remember that while the jungle and her creatures might seem scary at times, they are "all my relations" and support you and the planet. Your perspective broadens. Like the jaguar, you discover you can venture far from your familiar birthplace, exploring new territory, feeding yourself and your young, thriving in the lush primordial garden of the earth.

The people who dwell in the rainforest know that all beings are dependent on one another and are interconnected. You recognize that you're not alone and not meant to take an attitude of "I'll just look out for me."

HOW DOES PSYCHOLOGY FIT IN?

Psychology tells us that we can change our lives if we can change our minds. However, we spend tremendous efforts to change our thoughts only to find ourselves still stuck in habits and behaviors that hurt others and ourselves. Today we know that you can change your mind only after you change your brain; that is, after giving it the nutrients it needs for repair (not by medicating it with pharmaceuticals) and by creating a rite of passage or ceremony.

Earlier in the book, I shared a fire ceremony you can use to "burn away" toxic beliefs and be able to more easily change your mind and your brain.

A great benefit of psychology is that it helps us comprehend the mystery of our existence in a deep and authentic way. Yet we have often used it to excuse and justify to ourselves and to the world how our shortcomings are the product of our trauma or upbringing, and how our childhood is keeping us from who we could become.

Psychology helps us own our wounds and discover the gifts in them, and the lessons that life is offering us. We come to recognize the instincts of our ancient brains—which we've been learning about in earlier chapters—so that when they leap out unannounced and steer us toward unwarranted actions and emotions, we can invite them to a healthier, wiser expression. When we recognize fear raising its head again, we can choose to act from the higher brain, and respond with a loving and generous gesture.

The higher brain recognizes that whatever unconscious, deeply held beliefs you have about life, the universe will endeavor to prove you are correct. If you're sure the world is a frightening place, you'll find plenty of evidence that you're right. And you'll develop behaviors that will keep you responding to the world as if you're being stalked by a jaguar. If you believe you're unloved and alone, you will overlook opportunities that may be right in front of you. But when you upgrade your brain, you can entertain the idea that the universe is mysterious, engaging, and even magical. If you discover the universe is abundant and that you have resources ready to be accessed, your trust will be rewarded by evidence that this is so.

How do we draw a map that helps us spot unseen treasures and transform a mindset of scarcity into one of abundance? It's true that we can't simply wish away our fearful beliefs. Upon examining them, we can see that they are producing behaviors that are not serving us and may even be irrational. Yet they're encrypted in our neural networks and become habits. Physical and emotional challenges offer us opportunities to draw new maps, but we don't have to wait until we're facing a health crisis, an emotionally devastating event, or a seemingly unsolvable problem to change our navigational charts. These will begin to transform when we upgrade the brain's hardware and our hippocampus.

We can start today—and change our minds, as we change our brains.

The jaguar mode of awareness the Amazonians speak of can help you transform fear and anger into courage and love. As your brain becomes primed for transformation, you'll be able to recognize options you overlooked previously because you were "blinded by anger" or "frozen in fear" and unable to look around in all directions. Just because you don't see the answers you seek doesn't mean they aren't available to you. You will learn that like the jaguar in the jungle you have no predators, that you are loved and supported by Pachamama.

We start by recognizing our indestructible connection to Pachamama—the implicate order—and go from there.

New Paths, Focused Attention

Something as simple as a meditative practice allows you to create new neural networks that support the higher mind. Richard Davidson, professor of psychology and psychiatry at the University of Wisconsin School of Medicine, has been studying Tibetan meditators and found that their brains are wired differently from that of most people. When these monks were placed in fMRI machines and asked to meditate, their brains went quiet. They didn't respond with fear despite being inside a metal monster clanging loudly around them. They showed no anger or upset. The only regions in their brain that remained active were the frontal lobes, which are involved in joyous mystical experiences and in quieting the ancient M-brain.[7]

Like the Tibetans studied by Davidson, we all need a meditative practice that rewards us for installing neural networks in the higher brain. Even monkeys need this. In the 1990s, Professor Michael Merzenich performed a series of experiments at the University of California San Francisco, where he tapped the fingers of two sets of monkeys. When the rhythm of the tapping changed, one group was rewarded with juice for noticing and responding to the change. The other group did not receive any reward. After six weeks, the monkeys' brains were examined. The researchers found that the monkeys that received a treat showed profound differences in reward areas of their brain, while the other monkeys showed no difference whatsoever.

You can see from Merzenich's research why all those gold stars and prizes we give to our children are important, and why positive stimuli works so much better than threats or punishment to train the brain. Yet negative, judgmental comments about what a terrible student or person we are leave their mark on us. As Merzenich explains: "Experience, coupled with attention, leads to physical changes in the structure and future functioning of the nervous system . . . Moment by moment, we choose and sculpt how our ever-changing mind will work, we choose who we will be in the next moment in a very real sense, and these choices are left embossed in physical form in our material selves."[8]

Living on autopilot will not create the neural networks that enable you to experience the world magically. Even meditating, playing the piano, or bicycling on autopilot can't help you achieve your highest potential. We need to break the habits of judging people and situations by an old ruler of victimhood. Earlier, I said that you want to go from asking "Why is this happening *to* me?" to asking "Why is this happening *for* me?" You also want to change the habit of asking "What's in it for me?" to asking "What is for the greater good of all?" These practices, together with gratitude for life, are the essential ingredients for activating N-brain networks. And then we reinforce these higher order neural networks with gratitude!

In my own life, I've found that meditation is essential. Most everything you do can be a meditation practice if you have focused attention. By focused attention, I mean a relaxed attention that notices the birds singing and the sounds of people moving around in another room but not being engaged by them. In the morning, my first practice is to wash the dishes before my wife wakes up. Then, I get in a few minutes of quiet meditation before making a cup of strong coffee. I have never liked washing dishes, yet when I approach this chore with mindful attention, I break the mental dialogue about how disgusting the task is and how we should just eat from paper plates. Now, as an anthropologist, I've taken part in archaeological digs, and I have never seen fellow scientists happier than when finding a 3,000-year-old garbage dump and examining the leftovers of a Paleolithic dinner. I myself have been thrilled to discover prehistoric poop to take back to the laboratory to examine what ancient peoples ate. But day-old dishes? Not for me.

At first, I would say to myself, "Ugh. I should be working on my brain book." I would tell myself I would rather do just about anything else than wash dishes, especially after having people over. "What a waste of time!" I would think. My M-brain was rebelling. And then I decided to do the 4:4 breathing practice. As I began to tackle the dishes, I would breathe in, breathe out, focusing on the experience. "There's nothing more important than any other thing in the world," I would pronounce to myself. Then, one morning, to my surprise, I discovered I was looking forward to doing dishes. Well, kind of . . . At least I now had a spiritual practice instead of just a morning chore.

You too can install new neural networks, but you must be *focused and engaged*—infusing meaning and purpose into your actions—for this to happen. And they are anchored and activated by gratitude. It also helps break old habits of perceiving challenges. One way I do this is by playing the game of Scrabble. If you're unfamiliar with Scrabble, it involves creating words out of wood-letter tiles on the gameboard. You and a partner (or two or three) make words in crossword-like fashion, building off the first word placed on the board and trying to figure out how to make as many points as possible as you lay down tiles to add a new word to the board. One day, I decided to play with the board upside down so I could not rely on ordinary sense-making. I would have to shift my perspective. Then I began to scramble my letters on the table instead of laying them in a linear fashion on the small plastic stand. I would relax my gaze and allow words to leap out from the soup of letters before me.

To practice focused attention, try to think of things you already do every day—maybe changing a habit you already have (like washing the dishes). The good news is that even if you merely *think* about washing dishes, you get the same response in the brain as you get from actually doing them (even if you don't get the same response from your spouse!). World-class athletes know this. One of my students, an American Olympic skier, would mentally practice her runs in the downhill moguls race. Skiing the downhill moguls is one of the most challenging and demanding competitions in any sport: You navigate a course with a series of icy bumps, or moguls, while also performing aerial maneuvers. Skiers are judged on their technique, their speed, and the difficulty of their aerial maneuvers. As you can imagine, the event requires balance, strength, and agility, as well as the ability to make lightning-fast decisions and react to changing snow and ice conditions. The year that I assisted this Olympian with her training, she won the World Cup in Japan. Focused attention through visualization is that powerful.

And research supports the incredible brain-changing potential of visualization. Dr. Alvaro Pascual-Leone is a neuroscientist who conducted research comparing the brain activity of individuals who practiced playing the piano with those who had only imagined playing it. Pascual-Leone and his team measured the changes in brain activity in pianists who practiced a specific piano piece for five consecutive days, compared to nonmusicians who only imagined playing the same piece. They found that both groups showed similar changes in brain activity in the area of the motor cortex responsible for finger movement, but the changes were more pronounced in the group who had actually practiced playing the piano. This suggests that mental practice can have a similar effect on brain activity as physical practice. It's also a good reminder to apply spiritual practice to your everyday life.

It seems to take about 30 days to install new neural networks that will change your perspective of the world. We know this because in the early days of the space program, NASA conducted an experiment to study how astronauts coped with disorientation in space. Astronauts wore 180-degree-flipping goggles around the clock, initially causing anxiety and stress. However, after 30 days, their brains rewired, and something unexpected and extraordinary happened: Their world turned right side up again.

When we repeat a behavior with attention, the connections between neurons become stronger. This makes it easier for the circuit to activate in the future, leading to a quicker and more automatic response—the basis of habit formation. Through repeated activation, these neural pathways become more efficient at establishing behaviors, as the brain starts to perform these actions with less conscious effort. Additionally, the release of dopamine—the rewarding neurotransmitter—during pleasurable behaviors can reinforce these pathways, making our habits even more ingrained. This complex interplay between synaptic strength, neurotransmitter release, and neural circuitry underpins our daily habits. Take eating dessert, for example. Why would we want to ruin a nice, healthy dinner with a sugary treat? This may be because habits developed by ancient humans (still operant within us) who discovered that most everything sweet in nature was not poisonous, that it was safe to eat, make us associate a sense of safety with sweets. We want to feel safe before we retire to sleep. Neurons in our stomach sense the presence of sugar and communicate to our brain (through the vagus nerve) that all is well in the world (even as we are becoming prediabetic) and we can let our guard down.

We will not change long-standing beliefs despite being supplied with all the evidence in the world as to why they are not true. But we can change our behaviors through creative practice that installs higher-order networks and allows the ones in the M-brain to dissolve naturally from lack of use.

Whatever you practice in your mind and in your life will bear fruit in the world. The next task is to begin to practice something different. This is how the inventor of the sewing machine decided to place the hole of the needle in the head of the needle, as if a regular sewing needle were turned upside down. Seeing the world, nature, technology, and one another with different eyes can lead to breakthroughs.

Superforecasters and Intuition

It isn't only science-fiction authors writing about the extraordinary powers we can turn into reality when we awaken the higher brain. Secretive U.S. government agencies (the CIA and the NSA) are actively studying how to put these powers of the new brain to use. Philip E. Tetlock, a scientist at the University of Pennsylvania, heads the Good Judgment Project, which aims to study the accuracy of expert predictions in various fields. Since 2011, the project has recruited thousands of "superforecasters" from around the world to make prognostications on a wide range of political, economic, and global events. Elite teams of "superforecasters" were asked to predict future movements of military forces, placements of strategic armaments, and political hot spots around the world. Tetlock discovered that his elite teams predicted future geopolitical and economic events with more accuracy than analysts who had access to classified intelligence information.[9]

The American CIA has been interested in extraordinary human capabilities for decades. The Stargate Project, led by Hal Puthoff and Russell Targ, both physicists at the Stanford Research Institute in California (SRI), was a program that focused on the study of psychic phenomena, particularly remote viewing. The project was commissioned and funded by the U.S. government's Defense Intelligence Agency. It aimed to investigate the possibility of using an extraordinary ability called remote viewing for intelligence gathering and other military applications. (Remote viewing refers to the skill a person, known as a "viewer," uses to perceive distant or unseen targets, primarily Russian military installations, using extrasensory perception.) The SRI project produced a number of classified reports on the results of its experiments.

I was introduced to Dr. Targ in the 1970s when I was a graduate student working with Dr. Stanley Krippner. At that time, we knew that Dr. Targ was doing some kind of secret project that involved using "psychic" abilities to not only find Soviet nuclear missiles but even attempt to sabotage them in some way by interfering remotely with their electronics. I also met Dr. Targ's daughter, Elizabeth, who at that time was completing her training in psychiatry at Stanford University. Elizabeth and I became fast friends, and she traveled with me to Peru on several occasions to meet and work with the Indigenous elders. She told me that as a child she would have to guess the content of her Christmas and birthday presents before opening them, and that her father would challenge her to call the outcome of presidential elections, horse races, and other world events. After completing her medical degree, she spent years studying the power of remote healing, in which people would pray for the well-being of individuals who were not physically present.

Elizabeth's first study, published in the *Western Journal of Medicine* in 1998, involved AIDS patients who were randomly assigned to receive medical care and distant healing or standard medical care only. The study found that those who received distant healing had a significantly lower rate of hospitalization and death than those who received standard care alone.[10] Dr. Targ conducted many studies on distant healing, including a study of patients with advanced breast cancer, which found that those who received distant healing had significantly higher survival rates than those who did not.

In one of our Peru expeditions, Elizabeth and I conducted a small experiment with remote viewing. Elizabeth trained our participants to enter a quiet relaxed state, focusing on their breath, and to track into the future to determine the three colors and three geometrical shapes that she would be drawing on a sheet of paper that evening before dinner. To our surprise, many of us were able to accurately predict her choices—far more than would have been achieved due to chance!

Future tracking is one of the capabilities of the higher brain, which can use this skill to help us make decisions relying on more than only the facts before us. And if Elizabeth and the superforecasters and the Amazon elders are right, we can participate in selecting a future destiny we desire. Perhaps this is something that the higher brain does once we enter the quiet place of deep meditation. Who couldn't use a little more help selecting their destiny and preparing for a future of uncertainty and information overload?

The higher brain is excited to ride the waves of change, is interested in lifelong learning, and relishes questioning and discarding old habits. The resilience we need won't happen if our higher brain has been hijacked by the M-brain. Remember that the hippocampus is in the ancient M-brain, and when it's damaged, we resort to living on autopilot, falling into old habits and behaviors. We stop questioning the old and feel threatened by new technologies and change.

Fears about what problems may arrive with the coming tsunami of change can create stress, but as you'll learn in the next chapter, there are other stressors that wreak havoc on our brains. The more you know about the biology of stress, the easier it will be to understand why it's important that you not underestimate what the accelerated rate of digital innovation is already doing to your brain.

Key Takeaways:

We explored the power of limiting beliefs and ancient neural networks.

1. The higher brain, and its role in healing fears and traumas, dismantling outdated beliefs, and resolving chronic stress. Recognizing and healing unconscious beliefs can lead to a shift in mindset from fear to love and courage.

2. The necessity of recognizing when normal coping mechanisms are dysfunctional. Only the higher brain can recognize these patterns and promote self-honesty, ultimately leading to a shift in mindset.

3. The value of wisdom and adaptability in survival and evolution, highlighting the need to break repetitive behavior patterns and seek different solutions when faced with challenges.

4. The story of the journey in the Andes highlights how being in the flow with nature and being attuned and open to the guidance of natural elements can lead to fortunate outcomes.

Chapter 5

STRESS, BOTH GOOD AND BAD

In the West, mental and emotional stress has become as common as air, and we all seem to suffer from childhood trauma. Often, we try to manage these by self-medicating (from alcohol to mood enhancers to microdosing psychedelics) or pharmaceutically. One in six Americans takes an antidepressant or other psychiatric drug,[1] and it's no wonder. We are facing crises that are impossible to ignore if you have a news app on your smartphone, where "breaking news" is 24/7, reminding us of something else we can panic about. But stress and trauma are not only psychological. They are also biological. And they acquire a new significance in our postmodern world.

A Time of Exponential Change

In your great-grandfather's time, you could count on things remaining pretty much the same as they were during his grandfather's tenure on earth. Other than the discovery of America, which was doubted by many because it contradicted the obvious evidence that the earth was flat, the world didn't change much from one generation to the next. In fact, our brains had not had to deal with much novelty since inventing the bow and arrow 50,000 years earlier. But today, the power of computers and AI is doubling every 18 months. In a digital world, change is no longer incremental but exponential. We can no longer measure change occurring in decades, when a few weeks can turn the order of the world around, and we will know about it immediately.

Our M-brain believes that the world should still be changing gradually. In effect, predictable events don't evoke much of a response from hippocampal neurons, as there is no learning involved when what is happening doesn't contradict the predictive circuits in our brain. However, a handful of neocortical neurons in our N-brain get very excited with novelty and alarmed when there is a mismatch between the actual and anticipated events we encounter. Something is wrong, we decide. In reality, nothing is wrong with the world, but something *is* wrong with our brain's stale, dated maps of reality.

Our M-brain guided our lives for thousands of years when most of humanity lived in scarcity and hunger was rampant. We're not in the 1600s anymore, a time when the king or chieftain was a totalitarian ruler, most of us were serfs, and children fought over a piece of bread, yet we have epigenetically inherited the mindset of there being only "so many slices of the pie," and we better get our own. It's wired into the archaic maps in the hippocampus. This mindset will determine how successfully you will navigate the exponential changes in the decades ahead.

We think we are living in extraordinarily stressful times, but in reality, we are only bumping into the speed limit of our M-brain. For example, life in Europe during the Middle Ages was much more dangerous than it is today. Our medieval ancestors lived in constant threat of annihilation from neighboring armies and marauding thieves. A *National Geographic* article titled "What Made Oxford's Medieval Students So Murderous?" states in the opening paragraph, "The Middle Ages were a deadly time to be a student at the University of Oxford—they were roughly three times more likely to commit murder or be brutally murdered than other residents of the medieval English city."[2] No, it was not a carefree life in Europe back then.

In fact, we are living in one of the most peaceful eras humanity has known. Two centuries ago, most countries were led by dictators and autocrats. Now, most countries are democracies or on their way to becoming them. Challenging our M-brain's "scarcity circuits," the world today is moving toward increasing abundance for all. Already, technologies are offering a vast number of people the resources to live in comfort, have a future for themselves and their children, and not be trapped in a cycle of hunger, poverty, and despair. In the not-too-distant future, space mining—where we recover precious minerals from comets, and no longer have to be extracting them from our planet earth—promises to bring abundance to all. Breakthroughs including AI, biotech, robotics, and genetics are quickly democratizing our society and allowing everyone to have a slice of the pie.

Yet if this is the case, why are we so stressed and traumatized? Could it be because our analog brain is not comfortable with exponential change?

A Secret about Stress

In engineering, stress is a measure of how a material reacts to externally applied forces. If you place a load on a steel beam, it will resist, but if you overload it, the beam will give way—it becomes "the straw that broke the camel's back." Despite most humans being free of the hardships we experienced hundreds of years ago, unique modern stressors are overloading our brains. One culprit is the never-ending digital stimulation that is keeping our amygdala cranked up and our fight-or-flight system unable to reset itself. Having the alarm switch chronically in the "on" position has injured the hippocampus—for many of us it has shrunk to half its size, leaving us unable to turn challenges into eustress, a form of stress that's actually good for us (*eu* comes from a root word meaning "good").

We'll readily accept the stress of starting a new job, getting married, or having a baby because of the payoff. Eustress feels exciting and motivating. It might invite us to learn something new or cause us to become better at a task. For example, stage fright can turn into a better, more powerful performance. Every time I get ready to give a talk, whether to 10 or 1,000 people, I feel my shirt is a bit too tight around my neck, and I am certain I will forget the key points of my speech. After many years of speaking publicly, I have learned to welcome this moment, for it keeps me with a "beginner's mind" and open to discovering what is important in the moment. I have learned that nature abhors experts and that if I ever approach a speaking engagement overconfident, I will succeed in simply delivering facts and not bringing about the kind of positive engagement that is so valuable.

Just as your muscles will get stronger through exercise, the higher brain responds to creative challenges and eustress. But remember, stress has less to do with what you are doing than with how gracefully you are doing it. Challenges can push us to do things we didn't imagine we could do, to become explorers and inventors. But as we grow older, we often develop a "been there, done that" attitude. Few things excite us anymore. Yet give a wrapped Christmas present to a child and you'll see them bubbling with excitement at the mysterious gift hidden inside. With eustress, we can feel our pulse quicken and our hormones surge in a good way. Anticipation and excitement build.

I remember taking my son to the Bahamas on a special shark dive when he turned 15. It was to be a surprise, but he knew something was afoot when he saw the divemaster on the boat put on chain mail (the type that knights going to battle would wear). We had already suited up with our masks and fins, and each of us set up our scuba breathing apparatus. Little did I suspect that I would be the one to be surprised.

The divemaster was helping others in our group with their gear, and as I was ready, he indicated that I could jump into the water and meet the group in a few minutes at the bottom, 50 feet below. So, I made my way to the stern to the dive platform and prepared to enter the water, holding on to my mask with one hand and my tank with the other, ready to do a butterfly kick once I hit the water. Just then, I noticed five sharks swimming near the sandy bottom.

Yes, I'd signed up for this, but I had not consulted my M-brain, which switched on my fight-or-flight response immediately, and I felt a surge of adrenaline through my body. I quickly did the math: With 12 divers, there was less than a 10 percent chance of my being lunch. With only one diver, the odds changed dramatically.

And then I did the breathing exercise—the 4:4 breath—and my neocortex managed to quiet my amygdala. A surge of excitement ran through my body. I jumped into the water and descended slowly, still keeping an eye on the sharks, fascinated by these beings that have been on the planet for 350 million years and were now waiting for the divemaster and the frozen fish feast he was bringing. My arms crossed, I continued the 4:4 breathing as I descended past the level where the sharks were circling, fascinated as much by the changes in my brain and nervous system as by these creatures gliding above me that had only a reptilian brain. Suddenly, one swam very close, brushing against my face mask, and I reached out automatically to pet it. It wasn't interested. It had just come by to see if this being with the black wet suit was food, danger, or neither.

Signs That Damaging Stress Is Getting to You

The concept of harmful stress is not new. The ancient Egyptians believed that illness was caused by an imbalance in the body's "humors," the fluids that were thought to control emotions. The Egyptians believed in maintaining a balance between work and leisure and recommended exercise and meditation to help cope with the challenges of daily life. The ancient Chinese believed stress resulted from an imbalance in the body's "qi" or life energy and, if not addressed, caused disease. But the modern understanding of stress as a physiological response to challenging situations originated in 1936, when Hans Selye, a Hungarian endocrinologist, introduced the concept of "general adaptation syndrome" to describe the body's physiological response to challenges. Selye's model served as the foundation for much of the research on stress that followed. But it wasn't until the second half of the 20th century that the notion of stress became widely studied and its symptoms identified. These include digestive issues, overeating or undereating, fatigue, irritability, anxiety, and more.

When you're chronically stressed, you may find yourself losing interest in daily activities and not finding joy in what once gave you pleasure and isolating from friends and family. The damage chronic stress does to the brain, and specifically, to the hippocampus, is caused by inflammation. When microglia, the immune system of the brain, are activated by stress (whether emotional, physiological, or chemical), they release molecules called cytokines whose task is to signal the immune system to go into action. These molecules can metaphorically set your brain on fire—producing chronic inflammation.

Inflammation is beneficial when it's acute—a natural response of the body to injury, infection, or disease, and it typically lasts only a few days. This is what happens when a mosquito bites you (and the spot turns red) or when you scrape your knee. When your immune system responds, inflammatory molecules combat bacteria and help to repair injured tissue. When your body releases cytokines in the absence of illness or injury, chronic inflammation can last for months or even years. It's a common symptom in conditions like arthritis and AD.

This happens when cortisol, a potent anti-inflammatory (related to cortisone), comes in. Medieval warriors were helped by cortisol when they were injured on the battlefield, as cortisol releases sugar reserves that allowed them to fight on or flee. There are legends of warriors remaining in the battle after being struck by enemy arrows multiple times, thanks to the cortisol and adrenaline rushing through their veins. Cortisol also assists the hippocampus in forming memories that helped the warrior avoid future traps and dangers. Yet persistent cortisol production will damage the brain, even as short-term exposure has positive survival benefits. When we're unable to meet challenges creatively, when we are unable to put up a fight or run away, we end up freezing. Even if you are emotionally "frozen" in a marriage or a job you know you should have left years ago, your increased cortisol production will damage your brain.

Chronic inflammation causes us to age faster, which is why it is known as inflammaging. We all know people who suffer from innumerable -itis (inflammatory) conditions, from arthritis to bronchitis to colitis, gastritis, laryngitis, and tendonitis. As the years go by, our inflamed bodies become less able to deal with physical and psychological stressors. Little things will set us off and trigger a disproportionate rebuff or angry response. The accumulated damage in our brain furthers the decline of the immune system (known as immune senescence). You can be 40 years old with the immune system of a 75-year-old.

Toxic Buildup

Chronic stress is exacerbated by the toxic load in our bodies—pesticides, mercury, and chemicals such as dioxins and PCBs, for example. We know that many pesticides work by attacking the mitochondria (the cell's power centers) in insects considered pests. Imagine what these toxic chemicals do to our own mitochondria (which make up about 25 percent of the volume of a cell—and a single cell can have as many as 2,500 mitochondrion). As our mitochondria become less efficient, we lose muscle, which can begin as early as the age of 30. We know that mitochondrial dysfunction is at the core of Parkinson's disease. And research shows that exposure to pesticides such as rotenone, often sprayed on lawns and gardens and our vegetables, increases your risk of developing Parkinson's.[3]

The consequences of ingesting foods grown with those pesticides goes beyond increasing the risk of Parkinson's, as poor mitochondrial function is a hallmark in many diseases. We need to protect our mitochondria, for they are in charge of the death clock inside our cells, a process known as apoptosis (or cellular suicide). Our mitochondria protects us from age-related dysfunction and senescence through mitophagy, a powerful recycling process. Mitophagy helps break down the component proteins of old mitochondria, so that healthy new ones can use these building blocks to grow and develop inside neurons and all cells.

We have so many mitochondria-damaging toxins in our environment that even if we do our best to detoxify our bodies and brains, we are being poisoned daily by what we breathe, drink, and put on our plates. But not all toxins come from the outside world. Many toxins are produced in the body by the normal breakdown of spent hormones. Infections can also lead to the production of toxins, the by-product of the immune system's fight against bacteria or viruses. The body is meant to eliminate toxins through the liver, urine, feces, and sweat, but sometimes, it can't keep up with this job. When this happens we retox.

The liver aids in detoxification by breaking down and eliminating from the bloodstream toxins and other harmful substances including medication. But the liver cannot perform this function unless it has four essential elements: magnesium, zinc, vitamin B_{12}, and glutathione, an antioxidant you'll learn more about in Chapter 7: Reduce Free-Radical Activity, Support Your Mitochondria. Most of us do not consume sufficient avocados, nuts, and fatty fish to meet our minimum magnesium requirements, leaving us deficient. We're also often too low in the other three elements to be able to properly detox.

Upgrading your brain requires eliminating the toxins stored in brain cells, and if your liver can't eliminate these you will retoxify and become even more brain fogged than you were. As you'll see when you look at the program, in Chapter 11: The Grow a New Brain Program, I suggest you take these four nutrients as supplements. In addition, I like to take alpha lipoic acid, a brain detoxifier that can cross the blood-brain barrier and helps repair nerves, once or twice a week.

THE FINEST MITOCHONDRIAL INTERVENTIONS, BEST WHEN DONE TOGETHER

As I entered my 60s, I turned my attention to enhancing my mitochondria, the cell's energy factories that convert food and oxygen into ATP, our body's energy currency.

Imagine going from the beach to the top of Mt. Everest every five minutes. I am on the medical advisory board of a German company called Cellgym, which developed a device for maintaining mitochondrial health and energy production, essential for delaying aging. It alternates between providing oxygen-reduced and oxygen-rich air through a mask, simulating a climb from sea level to high altitude. I do this interval hypoxia-hyperoxia training (IHHT) two to three times a week for optimal mitochondrial function. It's been used by high-performance athletes—when you are at the top of Everest, aged and weak mitochondria die off, and a few minutes later when you are back at the beach the oxygen-rich air supports the genesis of new, young mitochondria. Cellgym is widely used in the United States and Europe in longevity centers for rejuvenating mitochondria, enhancing physical and mental performance, bolstering immunity, accelerating recovery, aiding weight loss, and stabilizing hormones. This is my favorite longevity device!

Our bodies are equipped with systems that repair and defend against aging, which poor diet, stress, and inactivity can disrupt. Mitophagy, the clearing out of broken and senescent mitochondria, is crucial for taking your brain health with you for the rest of your life. Certain plant products reset the kill switch in aged mitochondria so they can be recycled and replaced by new ones. Since neurons do not divide and replicate, the way they renew themselves is by replenishing their mitochondria. I am a big fan of the power of bacopa, lion's mane, fisetin, quercetin, pterostibene, and others to restore mitochondrial health.

You can learn more about these and other mitochondrial enhancers at my website, albertovilloldo.net.

Cool That Inflammation, Heal That Gut

To cool your chronic inflammation, you have to consider if it is being caused by a leaky gut. Given sufficient time and a strong enough inflammatory response, a leaky gut can lead to a "leaky brain." In other words, you'll have a brain that's on fire, awash in inflammatory molecules. A "leaky brain" happens when the tight junctions of the blood-brain barrier are penetrated by toxins and bacteria that have the potential to harm the brain. To extinguish the fire in your brain, you need to address the dysbiosis that's at the root of your leaky gut. You have to revisit your relationship to processed grains and gluten.

Around 10,000 years ago, grains became a dietary staple and we stopped eating a variety of the more than 50,000 edible plants available in nature. Our new grain-based diet was deficient in tryptophan, the precursor to serotonin. With increasing dysbiosis caused by the gluten protein, we stopped producing sufficient amounts of serotonin. The hippocampus began to atrophy, unable to repair without adequate supplies of serotonin. Learning and creativity suffered, and we ceased exploring the world. Our ancestors became sedentary farmers, followers of a new religion, where we asked God for our daily bread.

The American historian Jared Diamond, in his essay "The Worst Mistake in the History of the Human Race," argues that the discovery of grain-based agriculture was humanity's biggest blunder due to its damaging impacts on health, social structures, and the environment.[4] The shift from a hunter-gatherer lifestyle to farming led to population growth and the first towns, yet intensified social and gender inequalities, creating divisions of labor, wealth disparities, and the hierarchies and power imbalances evident in modern societies.

Our bodies and brains did not handle processed grains very well, and inflammation became a societal as well as a personal curse. Inflammatory politics and repressive religious fervor led to frequent conflict between neighboring villages and towns, culminating in the Crusades and the Spanish Inquisition.

From Stress to Adaptation

The Grow a New Brain protocol will help you repair a leaky brain with beverages and probiotics made in your kitchen laboratory. But you can't enjoy the creative N-brain until you deal with the damage caused by trauma. Our psyches, like the beam stressed by a heavy load, are stressed beyond tolerance. Our brains can only take so much of a toxic load of angry rebuttals, self-judgment, heavy metals, pesticides, and forever chemicals before their ability to resist the onslaught is overwhelmed.

In evolution, stress from a changing environment forces animals to find creative ways to adapt. It's what caused our ape ancestors to begin walking on two legs instead of four and protohumans to leave Africa to explore abundant lands elsewhere. Likewise, the personal challenges we're experiencing today can lead us—shepherded by the N-brain—to greater creativity and innovation. We know that while some people are devastated by trauma, many will experience post-traumatic growth that might never have happened otherwise. You can look at it this way: Everything you are living through is happening so you can discover something much greater, namely, a more successful strategy for crafting a meaningful life. As I mentioned earlier, you begin by asking "Why did this happen *for* me?" instead of "Why did this happen *to* me?" You are being invited to subscribe to the theory of the survival of the wisest rather than the hardiest.

Jonas Salk, whom I mentioned earlier as coming up with the idea of "survival of the wisest," was proposing wisdom as a cure to the ever-increasing internal stressors we are experiencing in the postmodern era. Fortunately, in the years since that dialogue I had with one of the preeminent scientists of our time, we have learned much about how we can reverse the damage done by stress.

When acute stress occurs, you find yourself geared up for a battle or a quick escape, and able to draw on increased focus and strength in a short-term crisis. However, stress can make it harder for the body to fight off infections and illnesses, as cortisol suppresses the immune system. And if you continue to experience anxiety and tension, unable to find creative solutions, you will develop chronic stress. Seldom does chronic stress result in creativity or learning a new set of skills, like short-term stress can help us to discover. To the contrary, it results in PTSD and denial/avoidance. We know that the M-brain can't differentiate between a painful experience that occurred 20 years ago and one that is happening right now in your life. This brain will superimpose the decades-old memory over the experience you are having today and choose the same dysfunctional solution it applied before. Instead of healing, you end up reinjured and losing your heroic attitude toward life. And when we stop being heroes, we become victims and feel shame.

THE DESTRUCTIVE POWER OF SHAME

According to the Abrahamic religions of Judaism, Christianity, and Islam, humans began life on earth in the Garden of Eden, where they first experienced shame. Anyone who grew up with this origin story has, to one degree or another, internalized the belief "I am ashamed." After Adam and Eve ate the forbidden fruit, they ducked into the bushes and fashioned leaves into covers for their naked bodies. When God asked, "Why are you hiding?" Adam responded, "Because we are ashamed." Our first ancestors were banished from Paradise, cursed to experience the punishments of hard work, death of the body, and pain in childbirth. Shame does not mean "I did something bad." That's guilt. Shame means, "I am bad. I am not a good person. I am not worthy."

In contrast, Indigenous cultures have origin stories about belonging to the earth and sky. The garden into which they were born still surrounds them, even as lumber companies are cutting it down.

Many of us have had to grapple with feelings of not being worthy. Shame, like other emotions, is not only a response to an event or a memory but also a reaction to your interpretation of what happened. In other words, it is not just what occurred that activates the brain regions associated with shame, but also your memory and self-judgment. People who experience shame have increased activity in the same brain regions that are activated by physical pain, which explains why shame can feel so painful.

When I was a graduate student completing my Ph.D. in psychology, I worked for many years with children from low-income families in a program known as Head Start schools. Many of the children came from homes where the father was absent and the mother had contemplated not keeping her child. With time, I began to notice that some of the children who had the most severe behavioral problems came from unwanted pregnancies. They had not been wanted while in their mother's womb, and I am convinced they had internalized that feeling as a damning personal judgment. It's as if somehow, the belief "I am not worthy" registered in their developing brains. Perhaps they had assumed the collective shame that haunts all of us born under the Judeo-Christian myth, which had been reinforced by their feeling within their mother's womb that they could be expelled at any moment from the only safe place they knew.

Shame is a collective feeling shared by all of us in the West. We can even think of it as our defining emotion. It is the cause of tremendous anxiety, and our sense of disconnection from the natural world seems to confirm our condition as outcasts from the Garden, concerned that we'll be "discovered" to be the impostors we believe we are. The concept of nature does not exist in Indigenous cultures. "Nature" refers to the diversity of flora and fauna, of forests and life-forms all around us, but does not include humans. The name does not even exist in Amazonian languages. When referring to the animals, the peoples of the jungles speak of their "relatives" and of "all my relations," and that includes the forests and rivers.

Shame causes physiological distress, and in response, we'll often launch an amygdala-based reaction of attacking others. We tell ourselves that "they" are the ones who do not belong, who are not like us, who are the unworthy impostors. The people of another race or country trying to take what is ours. We have to heal this original wound so we stop blaming others for our shame. That is, wrest control from the amygdala and turn control over to the N-brain, which helps us respond to life in a novel way, so we don't find ourselves stuck in shame and blame.

When Stress Originates with Trauma

Traumatic experiences in childhood often result in chronic psychological stress.

When I was 10 years old, we were living in Cuba in the middle of a revolution. One day, my father placed a loaded pistol in my hand and told me he was going away for "a while." I had heard nearby gunfire and knew there was fighting led by Fidel Castro, but I didn't realize my family was in great danger. We were upper-middle class—affluent compared to many of our neighbors, making us a target for the revolutionaries. My father was expected to attend nighttime meetings with local militia groups that would last for many hours. Before my father left, he told me that while he was away, I was to be the man of the house and protect the women of my family—my grandmother, mother, and sister. "If anyone tries to break in, shoot through the door!" he said.

For weeks, I worried about what to do if anyone showed up to harm us or steal the last of our food. One day, I heard a knock on the door. We weren't expecting anyone, and I began to shake in fear. Then, the knock turned to pounding—and kicking. Like a scared 10-year-old, I put down the gun that I had been clutching and went to the window, where I saw three men in military uniform. One caught my eye and saw the terror on my face. I froze. He turned to his comrades, and said, "Come on. There's no one here. Let's go." And they did.

That experience changed me. My childhood ended, and I became a very serious—and silently frightened—child. I had recurring nightmares of people breaking down our door, taking away my family members. Never shy before, I began to fear strangers. After all, I had no way of telling who was a "good guy" and who was a "bad guy." Years later, as a college student in the United States, I found myself tensing up and breathing shallowly whenever I saw a fellow student sporting a fashionable beard and mustache—a look I associated with Castro's troops.

Like many traumatized people, I buried the story of my pain. It didn't come back into my awareness until I realized that the frightened boy still lived within me and had been guiding many of my decisions and choices. I had been holding on to resentment toward my father for leaving us. The terror I had suppressed back then now poured into my mind and body. It took years for me to me begin embracing the frightened 10-year-old I had been and the stories I had created to feel safe and protect myself. Then came the challenging work of integrating the innocent 10-year-old, the one who believed that all the pain his family had experienced was his fault, that he was not good enough.

Many children grow up with the burden of trauma. Even when their childhood stories may not be dramatic enough to elicit gasps from listeners, they have lived experiences that imprinted themselves in their M-brains. Their unconscious beliefs leave the sufferers fearful of being abandoned, of never having enough food or love or money. They have brains that became wired by a survival instinct gone awry. The switch for their fight-or-flight response has become stuck permanently in the "on" position. Their M-brain is no longer helping them cope but rather damning them to being cast out of the mythic garden of safe childhood and a loving abundant world to live in.

You can see the domino effect: Stress causes physiological changes that rob us of our ability to have new experiences, hijacking the possibility of the new brain to creatively process input from the world, and our hippocampus struggles with learning new behaviors and ways of coping. We no longer know how to be like children newly discovering the world. As a result, we become calcified, stuck in our old ways. Our cortisol level declines and remains chronically low, so that instead of bounding out of bed in the morning we feel sluggish.

We can't see what's happening in the world today with fresh eyes and instead default to the old maps. I remember once, shortly after we had arrived in the United States, my grandmother refused to get on a "moving sidewalk" at the airport. "Sidewalks don't move," she goaded me. And she was right—if you consulted her internal map. The good news is that even if you have experienced trauma in your early years, you can upgrade your brain. You don't have to let the past determine your future. Your hippocampus can help you create a new map, exploring new potentials and identities instead of doing the same old, same old. You can create a new story for your life.

Who Are You, Really?

Once when I was on a hiking expedition in the desert of Canyon de Chelly in Arizona, Charlotte, an elderly medicine woman, taught me an important lesson about my "identity."

Charlotte was of Hopi descent, not related to the Navajo who lived at the bottom of Canyon de Chelly, where we were camped. I had prepared to visit her, bringing a hat to block the sun and enough water for probably three people, so worried was I about becoming dehydrated during the hike in the intense desert heat.

When I arrived at her summer shelter, I found her sitting outside under the shade of a cottonwood tree. We had met several years before during one of our annual expeditions to the birthplace of the Anasazi, but this was the first time we had a chance to speak with each other leisurely.

Charlotte asked me how I came to visit the land she called home, and I told her I was a newly minted Ph.D., leading a small group of students to visit the ancient cliff dwellings that the canyon is famous for. Her attentiveness was encouraging, so I began to expand on my biography.

"I've been living in America since I was a child," I said, "but I was born in Cuba. I escaped during the revolution with my mother, grandmother, and sister. My father was away when we got word that my family should leave as soon as possible." I went on to say that he was often gone, and soon, I found myself offering her my pop psychology analysis of how having an often-absent father had affected me and my life choices.

The elderly woman listened patiently, never interrupting. Finally, I paused and said, "So tell me about you."

She smiled and turned her eyes away from me toward the land.

"The red-rock canyon walls am I. The bright blue sky am I. The desert wind am I. The child on the reservation who did not eat today am I."

Then she returned her gaze to me, and I smiled awkwardly, embarrassed to realize that while her story was far simpler than mine, it was much more original and inspired.

We all tell stories of who we are, but do we know why we tell the stories we tell?

And how are those narratives working for us? Do they help us to be optimistic and creative, or do they keep us stuck in fear and worry, in the map created by our past suffering, explaining how we missed our chance at greatness?

We become the stories we tell.

Key Takeaways:

We explored themes related to the ancient M-brain and how it continues guiding our life and health.

1. We are the stories we tell, and those narratives can either foster optimism and creativity or keep us trapped in fear and scarcity.

2. The importance of upgrading our brains to break out of old patterns, becoming more secure by tapping into resources like wisdom, innovation, and positive emotions.

3. How *eustress,* the positive response to a new challenge, and how it can lead to increased excitement and a sense of exploration.

Chapter 6

UPGRADE YOUR BRAIN WITH BDNF

The ultimate brain builder might be an extraordinary protein called brain-derived neurotrophic factor (BDNF), which is like mother's milk for stem cells. To upgrade your brain, you want to ensure it has abundant BDNF on board. "Neurotrophic" refers to the ability of BDNF to regenerate brain cells and to minimize damage from free-radical activity and inflammation. BDNF also increases protein synthesis in neurons, the ability of brain cells to renew themselves by replacing all their component parts.

BDNF and Neurogenesis

BDNF supports neurogenesis—the maturation of new neurons—and protects existing neurons from degeneration, making it essential for optimal brain health. BDNF also promotes neuroplasticity, which is the brain's ability to reorganize itself by forming new neural connections. Deficiencies in BDNF have been linked to psychiatric disorders, including depression, schizophrenia, and neurodegenerative diseases like AD.

The higher-order neural networks facilitated by BDNF allow for creativity, imagination, and lifelong learning. BDNF protects mitochondria and can both shield the hippocampus and help it repair from damage. We need it for lifelong learning, but unfortunately, aging leads to a decline in BDNF, setting us up for growing duller and mentally fossilized as we age.

I remember as a boy of 11, when we had just arrived in the United States, my sister and I were alone with my grandmother at the house, and it was Halloween night. The doorbell rang, and my grandmother dashed to the window to see who was outside, then turned to me shaking, saying, "There is a crowd with sticks and dressed like skeletons!" None of us had heard of the strange custom of dressing up as goblins and demons on this night, so we turned off all the lights and hid in a closet. After the group left, my sister and I went back to watching television, but my grandmother would not come out of the closet for hours. While the cortisol and adrenaline washed out of my sister's and my systems, it was still coursing through our grandmother's. And her lack of BDNF made it difficult for her to ever enjoy Halloween . . . years later she would still lock the doors and turn the lights out even as she put candy by the entrance for the neighborhood children. She was not able to have a new experience replace her first encounter with ghosts and goblins.

Much as we might like to think of ourselves as mellowing with age like a fine wine, too many of us will turn into the stereotypical grumpy old man shouting at the kids to get off his lawn, or old woman bemoaning how her life should have turned out differently. Of course, we tell ourselves we'll never become that irritable, close-minded person, but too often, we can't exhibit the creative behaviors we swore we would adopt. Kindness and generosity elude us and old neural networks remain in the driver's seat after years of habitual conduct. But if we ensure that we have abundant BDNF, we can birth new neurons that override our most primitive fears, our negative emotional reactions, and damaging M-brain habits. You need new neurons like you need new skin cells, and BDNF helps strengthen the networks that allow us to look at the world in original new ways. When our hippocampus is repaired, we can embark on a journey of wonder and awe, with an imaginative and creative attitude toward life. By the way, BDNF also regulates energy metabolism in the brain and the body, determining how easily you can gain or lose unwanted pounds!

Science is still deciphering the complex puzzle of BDNF, and it appears that increasing BDNF production can even induce cancer tumor regression.[1] Daniel Radin and his colleagues at Stony Brook University School of Medicine found that increasing BDNF in the brain has the power to regulate the immune system to induce an antitumor response and reduce the activity of proteins that create resistance to chemotherapeutic agents. BDNF and the growth of stem cells and new neurons in the brain are another amazing example of epigenetics. It turns out we are not only what we eat but also what we think, and our moods and wisdom (and loving relationship with the world) epigenetically determine our health. This is called our exposome—the sum of what we've been exposed to and what we experience throughout our lives, including how you exercise, how you love and forgive, your level of stress, your microbiome, and the toxins in your food and water. More than 90 percent of your health or illnesses are determined by your exposome,[2] and it regulates how fast you age or remain youthful. All of these factors can help you increase BDNF, including consuming the omega-3 fatty acid DHA and eating five-day-young broccoli sprouts you will grow in your kitchen. Intellectual stimulation, social engagement, and staying mentally active, all of which are known to reduce AD risk, also increase BDNF levels. In the next section we'll look at how BDNF can keep your mind sharp and your mood up!

DHA for Boosting BDNF—and Preventing Alzheimer's

We worry so much about the fat around our waists that we forget about the fat in our brains. Brain fat is the good fat we want to keep. Sixty percent of the brain's dry weight is fat, and one-third of that is pure DHA! The retina in your eye is mostly DHA, and you need DHA to build the membranes around neurons that permit the transport essential nutrients in and out of the cell. A meta-analysis of 11 studies with 698 participants indicated that BDNF levels were significantly increased with omega-3 supplementation at doses of 1500 mg/day.[3]

DHA is also an efficient anti-inflammatory, helping extinguish the fire raging inside our brains. So where do we get the DHA that's so important for the brain? In utero, we got it from our mothers, and as infants, we got it through her breast milk (which is nearly 50 percent DHA) or today's enriched baby formula. (If you were fed infant formula in the previous century, it was made with inferior ingredients, with corn syrup or evaporated cow's milk, and you didn't get the DHA you needed in those formative months. This might help explain why all of us born before the year 2000 have behaved with such narrow-minded selfishness toward the earth.) After we are weaned, however, we may not have gotten the DHA we've needed all the years since. Most of us have brains that are DHA starved!

In the past, dietary sources of DHA were abundant—the fatty fish our grandparents ate were rich in DHA—but today, our fish are farm raised and fattened on a diet of corn. Fish can't make DHA from corn, only from eating the algae and smaller fish in their natural habitats.

The Indigenous people of the Pacific Northwest recognized the value of oils rich in DHA. The eulachon fish is also known as the candlefish because it's so oily that it can ignite when dried: the Nisga'a people used them as candles. What's more, First Nations peoples around Fishery Bay in Canada learned to extract the fish oil to create a DHA-rich "fat" that could be transported and stored without spoiling. The fish oil was so highly valued that it became a currency for people of the area. It provided fuel for the brain in the long winter nights, allowing individuals to find inner peace and wisdom that could carry them through the frigid months. A tablespoon of candlefish oil (which is still consumed by Nisga'a) provides more than 125 calories, and five ounces provide more than half of an adult's daily energy requirement. The Nisga'a are a peace-loving people who have long lived in harmony with nature. Is this because they have an unbroken brain?

The DHA supplements I recommend will help you upgrade your hardware. Your improved brain function will enhance all aspects of your life.

And fortunately we have the science to show it. The Memory Improvement with Docosahexaenoic Acid Study (MIDAS) studied the effects of DHA supplementation on older adults' cognitive function. The study recruited 485 healthy adults aged 55 to 80 years with mild memory complaints, who were randomly assigned to receive either a daily dose of 900 mg of DHA or a placebo for six months. The participants were tested for cognitive function using a battery of tests. Compared to the placebo group, the group that received DHA supplementation showed a significant improvement in working memory and executive function. (Executive function are skills related to adaptable thinking, strategic planning, self-control, memory, and more.) They also showed improvement in verbal memory and attention. The study concluded that DHA may prevent age-related cognitive decline.[4]

Even more impressive is a study conducted by Dr. Martha Morris and her colleagues at the Rush Institute for Health on the power of DHA to protect against Alzheimer's disease. They enrolled 815 healthy patients (aged 65 to 94 years) and followed them for nearly four years, at the end of which they found that 131 participants had developed AD. They discovered that participants who consumed fish once per week or more had 60 percent less risk of AD compared with those who rarely or never ate fish.[5]

Most Americans consume an average of 60 to 80 mg of DHA daily, which is far less than the recommended intake of 200 to 300 mg each day that's necessary for maintaining even basic brain function. The dosage that I use is closer to 30 times the average consumption of most people—2,000 mg daily. Occasionally, a student will ask me, "Isn't that too much DHA? Are there any side effects from such a high dose?" I like to respond that this is the amount of DHA you would get from eating a small portion of wild-caught salmon every night at dinner or a 15-minute "serving" of breast milk from your mother!

So, if you are wondering why your children—or you—continue repeating behaviors that are obviously self-destructive and not conducive to harmonious relations, the answer may be a brain that is starved for DHA. Without DHA, our brains cannot perform regular maintenance, much less the upgrade that we seek so we can discover solutions to our personal and collective challenges.

DHA regulates the activation of BDNF, and will activate the Nrf2 pathway—what I call the "Amazon pathway" because it was intuitively discovered by rainforest sages millennia ago—that switches off the genes for disease. (You'll learn more about this pathway, and other activators of it, in Chapter 9: Make Use of Powerful Pathways for Brain Health.) DHA and EPA in omega-3s are found in fatty, deep-water fish such as wild-caught salmon. EPA has been used as therapy for bipolar disorder and can help prevent coronary heart disease, reduce high triglycerides (fats in the blood) and inflammation, and lower blood pressure. I personally love the vegan version made from algae.

Curcumin for Boosting BDNF

Curcumin, the spice turmeric's main ingredient, has been used in traditional Chinese and Indian (Ayurvedic) medicine for thousands of years and possesses antioxidant, anti-inflammatory, antifungal, and antibacterial properties. (Earlier, I pointed out how many "anti" things there are in Western medicine. If you ask an Ayurvedic doctor about turmeric—known as the golden spice—she will tell you that it strengthens the body, relieves joint pain, and ensures longevity. No anti-anything.) Curcumin's ability to increase BDNF has attracted the interest of neuroscientists because villages in India, where turmeric is used in curry recipes, have only 15 percent of the incidence of AD as the United States does. Could that be due to curcumin's increasing BDNF production? Curcumin also activates the Nrf2 detoxification pathway, the "Amazon pathway" that silences the genes for cancer and dementia and protects mitochondria.

TIME-RESTRICTED EATING AND BREAKING YOUR FAST WITH HEALTHY FATS

To achieve maximum brain health benefits, you want to eat within a six- to eight-hour window and break your fast with healthy fats along with abundant greens. This allows your body to go into ketosis and detoxify during the remaining 18 hours when you are not consuming any food. I try to keep to this protocol four or five days a week, even when I am traveling.

Most mornings, around 11 A.M., I'll enjoy a green juice with the following ingredients:

1 cucumber, sliced

2 stalks celery, sliced

1 bunch baby spinach or kale (removed from stem)

1 small piece fresh ginger, to taste

¼ teaspoon *Rhodiola rosea* powder

¼ teaspoon bacopa powder

¼ teaspoon L-tryptophan powder

Juice of ½ lemon

½ green apple, cored and sliced

The green plants are loaded with signaling molecules (micro-RNAs) that switch on the genes for health. The herb *Rhodiola rosea* originally comes from the Himalayan highlands and improves endurance as well helping with attention span and clearing brain fog. *Bacopa monnieri* is a calming cognitive enhancer native to India. When laboratory rats exposed to chronic unpredictable stress where given *B. monnieri*, they began to produce abundant BDNF, resulting in neurogenesis and neuroprotection![6]

Midday I will prepare a feast for the bacteria in my gut, my microbiome. I know that when they are happy and healthy, so am I. This means a lot of fiber, so I prepare a large salad and a bunch of broccoli sprouts I grow in my kitchen. I will include asparagus sautéed in extra virgin olive oil and garlic, or a green pea and avocado hummus. I douse the entire meal in olive oil, for the healthy fats that will provide fuel for my brain.

In the midafternoon I might enjoy a smoothie made with blueberries and almonds and perhaps a half avocado (and occasionally a plant-based protein powder). Or I'll opt for a handful of roasted almonds or a bowl of blueberries. This will carry me to the early evening, when I might have something like an ancient grains tabbouleh or a roasted pumpkin with walnuts, with abundant olive oil. Once a week I may have a piece of wild-caught fish. And I avoid all dairy and eggs. All of these recipes can be found in my *Grow a New Body Cookbook*.

Healthy Fats

What are the healthy fats? At the top of my list are olive oil, avocados, coconut oil, and various nuts. The animal fats we're used to consuming (beef, pork, chicken, butter, milk, cheese) are packed with omega-6 fatty acids. In our not-too-distant past, we consumed omega-3 and omega-6 in approximately equal proportions. Today the standard American diet has a nearly 20:1 ratio of omega-6 to omega-3 fats. Excessive consumption of omega-6s found in beef are fueling an epidemic of cancer and heart disease. Yet, omega-6s in the right amount are beneficial for you. They help you maintain bone health, regulate metabolism, support your reproductive system, and boost skin and hair growth. So while omega-6 fats aren't "bad" or "unhealthy," we need to be sure we're not overconsuming them.

The Mediterranean diet has a good balance of healthy fats. This diet does not include much animal products, and it features foods rich in omega-3s, whole grains, fresh fruits and vegetables, garlic, fish, and olive oil. In all likelihood, this was the diet of your ancestors. They fueled their brains with healthy fats and ate little sugar: Most of their sugar intake was at the end of summer, when fruit was ripe. Your great ancestors stored the extra calories as fat to help them through the long winter. Similarly, humpback whales eat seasonally. Every year, they embark on an annual migration, with some journeying up to 16,000 miles round trip. During the summer months, they inhabit chilly, nutrient-rich waters teeming with krill, indulging in a feast. As winter approaches, humpbacks migrate to tropical waters, where they engage in mating rituals and give birth to their young. They will fast while in the warm waters, losing as much as half their body weight, living off their fat stores, and healing from skin cancer and other diseases.

The brain uses as much as 25 percent of your body fuel, and when your brain is running on fats, you begin to burn the calories around your waist. You have 50,000 calories stored in your body fat, which is a lot of energy compared to the 2,000 calories from sugar that are stored in your liver as glycogen. If you fuel yourself primarily with glucose, as we modern humans do today, you won't be able to break into your body fat's storage tanks! And if you eat excess animal protein, your body will convert it to fat around your waist.

The average American today eats close to 180 pounds of sugar per year, plus another 200 pounds of carbs in the form of pizza, pasta, and bread that become sugar as soon as they reach the stomach. A sugar-rich diet will clog your brain. Obesity and elevated blood sugar can be a fast track to AD, which is now being called type 3 diabetes.

To use your body fat, freeing up its energy, you must enter into ketosis: Your body and brain need to be burning a molecule called ketones, which your liver produces from your own fat stores. You'll achieve that by limiting your eating window to six to eight hours a day and breaking your fast with a green juice midmorning. On the Grow a New Brain program, you'll enjoy healthy fats from avocados, olive oil, nuts, and MCT oil. You'll also eat lots of vegetables and greens.

Sugars include fruits, which we too often eat in processed form (orange juice and jams, for example), and processed carbs (in the forms of breads, pastas, cereals, and crackers). The idea is to have your brain running on optimum fuel: healthy fats. The sweetness of life, it turns out, was never meant to come from sugar. It comes from freeing yourself of the tyranny of an ancient brain way past its expiration date and opening yourself up to learning, creativity, and bliss.

EAT MORE LIKE AN EARLY HUMAN

I like to follow the diet of early humans. Starting approximately 1.65 million years ago to around 200,000 years ago, the Acheulean period saw the development of stone tools, such as hand axes. The Acheulean diet consisted primarily of plant foods, including berries, nuts, and tubers, as well as occasional small game, fish, or food found from scavenging. Recent research on the benefits of eating like our ancestors has upended the meat-rich diets that were once so popular.[7] Like our ancestors, we have a hunter-gatherer genome, so we find it difficult to digest the processed grains that became part of our staple diet with the beginning of agriculture. And since we typically eat farm-grown berries bred for sweetness, we no longer get the benefit of the tart, hardy wild berries and their regenerative powers. This is why I buy frozen wild blueberries instead of the farm-raised varieties that are lacking the abundant Nrf2 activators you find in wild plants.

To Increase BDNF, Exercise

The word *exercise* may turn you off, but here's good news: Grueling, boring, repetitious exercise increases BDNF, but so does movement you actually enjoy.

A study at Harvard University showed that elderly women who exercised were biologically three years younger than the other women in the study and had a 20 percent lower risk of cognitive impairment.[8] High-intensity interval training (HIIT), like sprinting or running on a treadmill, produces much higher levels of BDNF than low-intensity exercise, like walking.[9] Yet both walking and stretching offer significant improvements in BDNF levels. The takeaway is to get moving, get active, walk, hike, stretch, and engage in some vigorous activity until you are out of breath for a few minutes each day to protect your brain for the rest of your life.

My favorite exercise is hiking—we have many hiking trails where we live. And I will do short bursts of faster walking and/or jogging, for 100 steps or so, enough to raise my heart rate, so I get the benefit of a mini HIIT exercise protocol.

Using the Power of Meditation to Increase BDNF

In the West, we think of meditation as a relaxation practice, used primarily for de-stressing. Indeed, it has these benefits, but it has others too. Seeing meditation only as a stress buster is like thinking that the sole benefit of jogging is to learn how to get places faster. Think of meditation as flexing the muscles of the brain. We exercise every other part of our body through movement. We exercise the brain through stillness, and meditation is the equivalent of HIIT for the mind. And best of all, meditation increases the production of BDNF as much as or more than any other exercise. Even among AD patients, the rate of progression of the disease is slowed in those who have meditation practices, probably due to increased BDNF production.

David Perlmutter, M.D., and I reached this conclusion, which we wrote about in our book *Power Up Your Brain*: "Meditation helps us visit the complex environment of the inner mind as well as the universal energy field. And, not surprisingly, this might well be the most powerful stimulant for BDNF production."[10]

Meditation is one of the most challenging practices I have ever attempted. It seems that you are just sitting there, doing nothing. Why is it so hard? When mental attention is turned inward and not to our to-do list, we are brought to a screeching halt at the end of the territory the M-brain controls. We reach a seemingly impassable fence: The M-brain continues to ruminate, remembering or planning, or it's tangled up in one emotion or another. On the other side of the fence is a peaceful field devoid of thought or emotion. But we don't know how to make it across. We search for the gate but find none.

The sages I met in the Amazon understood that on the other side of the fence lay the experience that we call gnosis. They know it as the "quiet place" because here, the mind is still. The brain goes into neutral, humming softly, while the only active area of the brain is the frontal lobes.

When Andrew Newberg, M.D., was the director of the Center for Spirituality and the Mind at the University of Pennsylvania, he used brain imaging techniques to examine the brain of meditators. In his book *How God Changes Your Brain*, Newberg describes how meditation enhances activity in the anterior cingulate cortex (ACC), a structure that bridges the two brain hemispheres. The ACC regulates empathy, intuition, and compassion, traits that we associate with spirituality, orchestrating signals between the amygdala and the frontal lobes. Newberg calls the ACC the "God brain."

The ACC can be thought of as the peacekeeper in the brain. While the amygdala might be in a "take no prisoners" mood, the ACC is interested in making friends and finding ways to collaborate.

Once the amygdala responds with anger, communication to the "God brain" is shut down. Newberg states, "Anger interrupts the functioning of your frontal lobes. Not only do you lose the ability to be rational, you lose the awareness that you're acting in an irrational way."[11] When your frontal lobes are offline, you're no longer able to hear your spouse make a point. You're too busy waiting for your turn to explain why your point of view is the right one.

Newberg treads fearlessly where few have dared to go. He makes the bridge between neuroscience and spirituality. He states, "We believe that there is a coevolution of spirituality and consciousness, engaging circuits that allow us to envision a benevolent, interconnecting relationship between the universe, God, and ourselves."[12]

Chilling with the ACC

When the hippocampus is upgraded, your brain can begin to craft new maps that find opportunity where before you only perceived danger. Change and innovation don't cause fear and paralysis anymore. The brain will be sending signals to the higher circuits so we can engage the world creatively. When the signal is sent to your higher brain and the ACC, the message is "Chill, dude. Look at the rosy side!"

The ACC is engaged during immersive study, meditative and contemplative practices, prayer that involves deep reflection, and experiences of transcending one's limited self and merging with a higher power or with the cosmos. When the ACC is on, you are free of primitive fears about survival and safety and experience life as a journey like that of the hummingbird.

Hummingbird Perception

If you're stuck in survival mode, getting through the day is going to take all your energy. However, when you discover you don't have to fix all your problems this afternoon, and that the universe has your back, you can begin to experience what Amazon peoples call hummingbird awareness. Defying all expectations, this tiny creature can fly for thousands of miles during its annual migration from

Brazil to its nesting place in Canada in the late spring. It can't see past the horizon, but it trusts in its journey. It doesn't freak out about the uncertainty of life.

The courageous traveler within you can soar when you surrender to the mystery of the wind and the unknown. You can do this even if it frightens you. With the ACC guiding you, you can immerse yourself in the womb-like darkness of the realm of possibility, exploring places beyond the map created by your culture, by memories from childhood, or from buried ancestral trauma.

Meditation will awaken the ACC and prevent you from identifying with the good or not-so-good experiences you are having. It frees you from feeling trapped and overwhelmed by your emotional state. When the ACC is engaged, and we're witnessing what we're experiencing rather than simply having an experience, we're able to recognize how temporary our moods and feelings can be. We understand that "this too shall pass."

I remember one night during a ceremony in the Amazon after I ingested a glassful of the visionary vine ayahuasca. In my visions, I was trapped in a tangle of roots and called out to the shaman to come and help me. He quietly observed that this was not a place "out there" but rather within—a mirror of my own mind. At that time in my life, I was in a very difficult relationship and could not disentangle myself. My hallucination was actually the reality I was living. At that point, I stopped struggling with the roots that were nearly strangling me and felt the higher brain take charge, offering me an understanding of my dilemma.

As I congratulated myself for having woken up from this harrowing vision, suddenly, the roots turned into snakes. I do not like snakes, even though I have admired boas in the jungle. Now I was panicking.

"It's my amygdala taking over," I said to myself, yet this knowledge brought me no comfort. Then I realized that the snakes were not suffocating or binding me; I was able to wiggle free and find a place of peace. The snakes had shown me how to be fluid and flexible and not rigid and demanding, as I had become in that relationship—one I was soon able to leave with gratitude instead of anger and resentment.

The ACC leads you to unexplored territories, where you can become enthusiastic about your life again and look in the mirror each morning to greet someone whose potential you have yet to discover.

Meditation awakens the ACC. Functional MRI scans of the brains of individuals who regularly practice meditation reveal distinct wiring patterns in contrast to non-meditators. Meditators' brains show heightened activity in the ACC in their frontal lobes during the states they refer to as samadhi. According to the Dalai Lama, achieving enlightenment requires freedom from destructive emotions and repetitive behaviors. This is facilitated by the ACC's capacity to quiet the amygdala, allowing for the experience of generosity and compassion and not only pouting and selfish behavior.

Upon activating the ACC you begin to override the M-brain's circuitry for fear. When that happens, the pursuit of happiness through other people or "things" becomes uninteresting and unnecessary, as happiness grows naturally. For the frontal lobes, happiness is not a product of luck or the toys you own; it arises from gnosis, from wisdom.

Intellectual Stimulation

There seems to be a direct relationship between educational level and risk for AD: The higher your education level, the lower your risk. AD typically begins 20 to 30 years before you are diagnosed, and prevention needs to begin decades earlier as well.

I imagine dementia as a storm slowly eroding a once vibrant city, the brain. At first, the storm's effects are barely noticeable: a few signs misplaced, some streets slightly harder to navigate. Over time, however, the storm intensifies, tearing down bridges of memory, flooding pathways of thought, and crumbling the houses of identity and skill that took a lifetime to construct. Landmarks that once were a testimony to a person's knowledge and relationships become obscured and then lost, leaving thoughts, memories, and personalities disconnected and isolated. Just as a city might struggle to function amid the chaos of a natural disaster, the brain under the siege of AD loses its ability to perform the tasks it once managed effortlessly.

You can begin with your daily dose of DHA.[13] This is one of the best investments you can make. And you can also seek intellectual stimulation, especially now that we are outsourcing our brains to our digital devices. We don't use maps anymore (we have a GPS— remember using a map to navigate?) or need to remember telephone numbers or directions. We need to exercise our brains as much as or more than we exercise our bodies.

As you do the Grow a New Brain program you will notice how your memory improves—today I have near photographic memory, yet when I was in high school and college and eating the typical SAD diet, I could hardly remember what my teachers had taught the day before.

Western Medicine Meets the Medicine of the Amazon

I first met David Perlmutter, M.D., author of best-selling books like *Grain Brain*, when his wife, Leize, who had read my books, suggested to David that they join me on an expedition. The trip involved hiking to Ollantaytambo, the start of the Inca Trail to Machu Picchu. As we hiked up the mountain along the ancient stone pathway crafted by the Inca some six centuries ago, the silence was broken only by the sound of a flute.[14] I had made this climb many times, and it is a challenging hike. Like many who aren't acclimated to the elevation—the Perlmutters were living 10,000 feet lower, in Florida—David experienced lightheadedness and shortness of breath. Before he could reach for his altitude sickness medication (acetazolamide) in his backpack, our Andean guide offered him some coca leaves and instructed him to chew them. Sure enough, the plant's effect was nearly immediate and quite potent. David's interest in power plants and the sages who know how to work with them was sparked. We would develop a friendship that involved many conversations and explorations of Indigenous healing, which eventually led to our collaboration on our book *Power Up Your Brain: The Neuroscience of Enlightenment*.

After the trip to the Andes, David returned to his medical prac- tice in Florida, cognizant of a wisdom that had been maintained and passed down through generations of elders. It was a wisdom that could do more than cure a mild case of altitude sickness. In David's words: "It was becoming clear to me that, overwhelmingly, the patients who achieved the most profound recoveries were those engaged in some form of meditative or spiritual practice."

Key Takeaways:

We explored various themes related to brain health.

1. The importance of consuming DHA to lower the risk of Alzheimer's.

2. The importance of intellectual stimulation, learning new skills, and having community with people who encourage creativity and imagination.

3. The significance of breaking down body fat through ketosis and burning ketones for brain and body energy.

4. Recommended dietary changes to reduce sugar and processed food consumption and instead focus on healthy fats, vegetables, and greens.

5. The benefits of following a diet similar to that of early humans, emphasizing plant foods and eating animal protein only occasionally.

Chapter 7

REDUCE FREE-RADICAL ACTIVITY, SUPPORT YOUR MITOCHONDRIA

By this point, you may be thinking this book is a little heavy on the science behind the Grow a New Brain program. I'm interested in offering you information that will help you take control of the destiny of your brain. To upgrade your brain, you must arrest the damage being done by free radicals. Aging mitochondria in your brain (they grow old on average after 10 to 12 days) produce free radicals—the by-product of inefficient combustion—like an old car burning low-grade fuel. Free radicals damage these power plants and act like terrorists. They steal an electron from another molecule to stabilize themselves, which makes the other molecule unstable and turns it into an electron stealer too. The result is oxidative stress, which damages your cells, tissues, and organs. Oxidative stress in your body is like the oxidation you see when an apple slice sits out too long and turns brown or a copper pipe exposed to the elements turns green. Oxidative stress plays a major role in the onset of depression.[1]

Free radicals accelerate aging and cause you to develop age-related diseases. (The theory of free radicals was first proposed by Dr. Denham Harman, a biogerontologist, who explained how antioxidants "quench" free radicals.) To reduce free-radical activity, you need antioxidants, which sate the terrorists, so they stop stealing electrons from other cells.

When our mitochondria are sick, we don't have energy. We have a dozen different reasons for how tired we feel, yet it all comes down to old and exhausted mitochondria—because remember, they are the energy factories in the body. Mitochondria also control the death clock, telling old, worn-down cells they need to die. When mitochondria are damaged, cells no longer know they need to die, and "zombie cells" build up in the brain. And when this happens you become sluggish, you only wake up after two cups of coffee, and you are shocked when you look in the mirror and see the new wrinkles in your face because young skin cells rich in collagen have not replaced the aging ones. And imagine what's going on inside your brain!

Mitochondria have their own DNA, different from yours, organized in a ring like that of bacteria. (You can think of them as friendly bacteria that exchange energy for a warm place to live.) The DNA in mitochondria are susceptible to damage from oxidative stress, as they lack robust repair mechanisms like those of our own DNA. Serotonin, which the pineal gland converts into melatonin, repairs DNA coding errors, functioning like a grammar and spellchecker to ensure we are regenerating cells without any spelling mistakes. Melatonin is the principal repair system for the mitochondria in our brain. Imagine what happens when we lack sufficient serotonin. Not only are we unable to produce the bliss molecules and live in the "flow" but also damaged mitochondria lose their ability to divide and begin to release inflammatory molecules that eventually lead to dementia. When mitochondria are unable to divide or to die, they become senescent, zombies that are neither living nor dead. Senescent cells are covered in more detail in Chapter 10: Arm Yourself for the Zombie Invasion: Eliminating Senescent Cells with Plant Medicines.

Mitophagy is a specific form of autophagy, a recycling process unique to mitochondria. The term *mitophagy* combines *mito*, from *mitochondria*, and *phagy*, meaning "eating," the process by which cells digest damaged mitochondria. This mechanism helps maintain a healthy population of mitochondria by recycling those that are no longer viable, preventing the accumulation of damage that makes cells become aged and senescent. This is why I love the brain nutrients that I mentioned earlier, because they support mitophagy and mitogenesis, the growth of new mitochondria in the body and brain.

The problem is that if you are over the age of 35, your production of the free-radical scavengers like glutathione and SOD (superoxide dismutase) will have diminished and be near zero. You won't be able to prevent your mitochondria from becoming damaged by free radicals.

Your ability to produce these antioxidants comes to a dead stop because of an ancient biological program preserved across all mammals that optimizes repair for the young. Biology wants to ensure youth can breed successfully and their offspring can guarantee the continuation of the species. This is nature's way of ensuring you don't live forever. After the age of 35, you can get antioxidants from foods and supplements, but these don't provide you with enough to keep up with the damage continually being done to your brain. You would have to eat the equivalent of 40 pounds of berries daily to quench all the free radicals your senescent mitochondria produce as a by-product of burning oxygen. And while you can get oral glutathione supplements, our guts destroy it (unless it is liposomal or nano encapsulated) before it can get to the bloodstream or the brain. Fortunately, we now know how to upgrade our biology to restart the manufacture of our own SOD and glutathione—which you'll learn about in Chapter 9: Make Use of Powerful Pathways for Brain Health.

Glutathione, the Superstar Antioxidant for Protecting Your Brain

Glutathione is a superstar antioxidant that is vital for repairing mitochondria, protecting the hippocampus, and detoxifying the brain. That's because beyond being a star antioxidant, it has a big sulfur molecule that helps transport toxins out of the brain. As if those functions weren't enough, glutathione also supports our immune system. Produced from ingesting foods rich in sulfur (like garlic), glutathione makes its way to our brain, easily crossing the blood-brain barrier. Recently, we've learned that neurons called astrocytes (named after their starlike appearance—*aster* means "star") can also manufacture glutathione.

Damaged mitochondria in senescent cells are responsible for many of humanity's ills, for they permit waste products of metabolism to build up in tissues, resulting in dozens of ailments, including fibromyalgia, a painful disease whose female sufferers outnumber male sufferers by a ratio of nine to one.[2] Too often, fibromyalgia's symptoms are dismissed by as being "all in your mind." In no small part, that reflects the medical system's long-standing dismissal of women's complaints, especially regarding pain, as being the product of "hysteria." (*Hysteria* and *histrionic* both come from the Greek word for "uterus"—in other words, too often, uterus-owners have been seen as crazy women making up their symptoms.) Note that when pharmaceutical companies realized that designing a drug to treat fibromyalgia could be profitable, the disease started to be seen as genuine.

MIGHTY MITOCHONDRIA AND THE FEMININE LIFE FORCE

The bias against women with mitochondrial dysfunction that takes the form of fibromyalgia—a very real and painful condition—is ironic given that the origin of human mitochondria is the mother's bloodline. Let me explain.

When I first met David Perlmutter, we started talking about plants that help repair the brain, and I mentioned that Amazon peoples believe we must restore the feminine life force for the sake of the planet and ourselves.

"Yes," David said matter-of-factly. "The mitochondria."

I stared at him in surprise. Of course! The mitochondria links ancient wisdom traditions with modern neuroscience. Mitochondria, you see, are within every cell, acting as its power generator—its life force, you could say. And we inherit our mitochondria from our mothers. Our mitochondrial DNA can be traced back to the first human mother, "Mitochondrial Eve," who appeared in Africa around 150,000 years ago. Her legacy can be found in our bodies today in the mitochondria in every cell. Not a single bit of mitochondrial DNA comes from your father's side. I am convinced that your health span and life span are largely influenced by your mother's side, from whom you inherited your "life force."

Glutathione turns out to be mitochondrial-protective. And while our bodies can create it (at least before biology deems us old and useless in our mid-30s), glutathione can also be produced in the laboratory. In fact, intravenous glutathione is used as an emergency treatment for acetaminophen overdose. David began using glutathione IV therapy on his fibromyalgia patients, with great success. And one of them had a response that shocked David. As he said:

"One September afternoon, I had the opportunity to evaluate a patient who, unfortunately, not only had fairly advanced fibromyalgia but Parkinson's disease as well. The latter had compromised his ability to walk to the extent that he was wheelchair-bound. We moved ahead with our newly discovered treatment for fibromyalgia and administered glutathione into his vein. What happened next forever changed my practice of medicine. About 20 minutes after the injection, this patient got out of the wheelchair and began to walk around the office.

"Italian researchers had, just one year earlier, demonstrated dramatic and long-lasting improvements in Parkinson's patients who received intravenous glutathione. The researchers reported, 'All patients improved significantly after glutathione therapy, with a 42% decline in disability. . . . The therapeutic effect lasted 2–4 months. . . . Glutathione has symptomatic efficacy and possibly retards the progression of the disease. And yet, perhaps because it was not a patentable drug, no one had gotten the word out to the tens of thousands of neurologists who treat Parkinson's patients every day.'"

Many people, including me, lack one of the genes to manufacture glutathione, so we do not produce enough of this free-radical scavenger to combat oxidative stress. I take 2,000 mg of glutathione IV every two weeks. You don't have to get intravenous glutathione injections to ensure you have enough of this superstar antioxidant. You can take N-acetylcysteine (NAC) in supplement form or eat NAC-containing foods such as nuts, cruciferous vegetables, spinach, carrots, and broccoli, as our guts absorb these building blocks of glutathione well. NAC, by the way, is a rock star for helping resolve long COVID. The best way to ensure you have sufficient glutathione is to make plants central to your diet.

While it's very important to reduce free-radical activity and support your mitochondria, you will also want to heal your gut so it produces abundant serotonin—not just for good mood but also to upgrade your brain. We'll look at that next.

Key Takeaways:

We explored mitochondria and free radicals and their impact on our brains.

1. The impact of mitochondrial dysfunction on conditions like fibromyalgia and Parkinson's disease, and the role of antioxidants in mitigating free-radical damage.

2. The connection between mitochondrial health, energy levels, aging, and age-related diseases.

3. Melatonin as a mitochondrial protective and its potential therapeutic application.

4. Mitochondria's role as the power generator in cells and its influence on energy levels and aging.

5. The link between mitochondrial dysfunction, conditions like fibromyalgia and Parkinson's disease, and the importance of waking up our dormant antioxidant systems.

6. The impact of free radicals and oxidative stress on cells, aging, and age-related diseases, and the importance of antioxidants in combating these effects.

Chapter 8

HEAL YOUR GUT SO YOU HAVE SUFFICIENT SEROTONIN

Serotonin is a ubiquitous compound. It's found everywhere in nature. In the plant kingdom, serotonin regulates flowering, photosynthesis, and growth. In fungi, it governs cell differentiation. In the animal kingdom, serotonin serves as a neurotransmitter, facilitating the transport of signals between nerve cells. The discovery of serotonin in every species, from invertebrates to humans, suggests that its role in regulating many biological processes has remained conserved throughout millions of years of evolution.

Serotonin is called the "feel good" molecule because it lifts our mood and helps us feel deserving of happiness and inner peace. You experience decreased anxiety and increased feelings of well-being. Low serotonin is linked to depression: Research at Rockefeller University looked at the postmortem brains of patients who had suffered from depression or anxiety. They discovered these brains show damage in areas that are strongly influenced by serotonin—and they note that selective serotonin reuptake inhibitors (better known as SSRIs) are the medications most commonly prescribed to address anxiety and depression.[1]

SSRIs prevent the reabsorption of serotonin into the neuron, thereby flooding the brain with serotonin. The SSRI-induced serotonin "bath" triggers the production of stem cells in the hippocampus. Curiously, you need to take SSRIs for six weeks before their effects become obvious—the exact amount of time that it takes for the hippocampus to grow new neurons from its bank of stem cells and begin to repair itself!

In addition to needing serotonin to renew our brain and uplift our spirits, it helps keep food moving along our gut as we digest it, a process known as peristalsis. It also helps control appetite and the sensation of fullness and satiety. In the hypothalamus, the brain region responsible for managing hunger, serotonin serves as a natural appetite suppressant. When serotonin levels are depleted, you can experience ravenous appetite and unexpected weight gain. The comfort foods we seek when we're feeling anxious or sad tend to be high in sugar and give us a short-term "serotonin high" that can exacerbate a vicious cycle of mood swings and compulsive-eating habits.

In the last decade, we have discovered that the brain and the gut are always speaking to each other—with serotonin facilitating this two-way conversation along the gut-brain axis. The axis includes a network of 100 million neurons in the walls of the GI tract, from your esophagus to your anus, and connects your stomach and intestines to your ancient reptilian and M-brain via the vagus nerve, where information flows bidirectionally between them. With all those neurons, it processes more information about the environment than the brain in your head—and all of it from the food you eat and the water you drink.

The microbes in your gut play a big role in making sure the gut-brain phone line works properly. They manufacture serotonin from tryptophan found in food, giving your mind clarity or creating brain fog if there is not enough tryptophan. Without abundant serotonin in our brains, we are miserable and grouchy—and more likely to develop dementia.[2]

You originally acquired your gut flora from your mother during birth, as you traveled through the birth canal. If your mother's biome had been ravaged by antibiotics, or if you were delivered through C-section, you were born lacking diversity of your microbiome. As you grow older, having fewer species of gut microbes will cause health problems. And recent research shows that people suffering from long COVID, with enduring symptoms like brain fog, fatigue, or memory loss for months or even years after their initial COVID-19 infection, have a reduced level of serotonin.[3]

One thing's for sure: A well-functioning gut supports higher-brain abilities.

Serotonin, Melatonin, and Sleep

Our sleep cycles are regulated by melatonin, a hormone manufactured from serotonin. Today, most of us don't have the serotonin levels that we need to sleep soundly, rest deeply, and renew and repair the brain. Melatonin sets our bodies' clocks. It's what allows the body to respond to darkness with the message, "It's time to turn in." Melatonin also increases the expression of the p53 gene, which is involved in managing cell growth. When melatonin nudges it, the p53 gene can do its job inhibiting the growth of tumors and the spread of unwanted cells.

Our internal biological clocks are set by sunlight, as they have been for millions of years. The blue sky and the first rays of sunlight in the morning shut down the production of melatonin and trigger a burst of cortisol that helps us bound out of bed with gusto (ideally!). Orange-red light, like that that of a campfire, will do the opposite, increasing melatonin production and making us drowsy. Remember that the world was lit only by fire for millions of years and our internal clocks—our circadian rhythms—were set by the blue sky and the rising sun and by the evening campfire or candlelight.

Today, even if the sky is overcast, the natural light will set your biological clock to the dawn. Even if your eyes are closed and you are fast asleep, the morning light will be registered and nudge you to wake up.

YOUR SLEEP CYCLE

Pigments in the eye known as melanopsin are sensitive to light and send signals to the hypothalamus, the body's "master clock" that regulates the circadian rhythm. The hypothalamus uses this signal to synchronize the body's clock with the external light-dark cycle and regulate your sleep-wake rhythm, body temperature, and hormone release. And most important, it sets the clock for melatonin production 16 hours later! Melanopsin is so sensitive that it can detect blue light from your smartphone while you are lying in bed in a darkened room. Your brain, believing that the sun is ready to rise, will wreak havoc on your sleep cycle. Your internal clock that controls many physiological processes over a 24-hour cycle will be set to a time zone you are not in!

If you want to reset your sleep cycle, get some early morning light, such as the sky-gazing exercise on page 119. Even looking at the horizon on a cloudy day will do the trick. However, if you don't have sufficient serotonin, your pineal gland won't manufacture the melatonin you need to rest, sleep, and repair damaged DNA. (Melatonin's role in the latter has earned it the name "the guardian of the genome.") I keep an LED panel—commonly known as a grow light, with blue LEDs—in the bathroom and turn it on in the morning to help set my biological clock during the winter. And this is an effective treatment for seasonal depression, common during shorter days and less sunlight of winter.

Lack of quality sleep harms your brain. While you sleep, when your neurons are not trying to make sense of the chaos in the world, your brain will shrink by 20 percent, allowing cerebral spinal fluid to flush away toxins and cellular debris.[4] When you are not sleeping well, your brain can't wash away trash like it's supposed to, and becomes inflamed, awash in excess cortisol that damages the hippocampus. The brain struggles to capture events into long-term memory, and we wake up in the morning with vague recollections of confused and chaotic dreams.

When your serotonin levels are low, you have difficulty falling asleep and remaining asleep. You'll wake up feeling fatigued and irritable. This will make you want to activate the brain's reward system—read "screen time" on your favorite digital platforms—to release dopamine from the "reward center," creating a pleasurable sensation and reinforcing your digital habit. As your dopamine levels decrease a couple of hours later, you find yourself returning for more, sometimes even reaching for your phone late at night when you awaken and can't fall back asleep, further disrupting your sleep cycle.

A friend was sharing recently how she took a two-week break from electronic devices but found herself in the first few days reaching for her smartphone and cradling it in her hands even though it was turned off. The addiction to our digital devices is now wired into our brains!

MY FAVORITE SLEEP AIDS

Andrew Huberman is a professor of neuroscience at Stanford University. We met when we were both presenting at a summit at the beautiful Six Senses Resort in Kaplankaya, Turkey, where I hold an annual weeklong Grow a New Body retreat. A scientist, he approached me after my presentation, where I had shared the missing link between neuroscience and ancient Indigenous wisdom. Our conversation over dinner turned to ayahuasca, the visionary vine of the Amazon, and its similarity to serotonin. I asked Andrew about sleep and circadian rhythms, being that both of us were on California time, nine hours different from the time in Turkey. The body can become very disoriented when you feel ready for a glass of wine at 9:00 in the morning!

Andrew shared his favorite sleep aids, below.

Magnesium threonate—2,000 mg
Apigenin—50 mg
L-theanine—200 mg
Myo-inositol—1,000 mg

I occasionally add 100 to 200 mg of 5-HTP to the mix to boost my serotonin levels during the night. But be aware that taking 5-HTP too often can result in a "crash" when you stop.

The body needs magnesium for more than 400 chemical reactions, and most Americans and Europeans are magnesium deficient. Magnesium threonate goes through the blood-brain barrier and raises magnesium levels in brain cells. Apigenin is found naturally in many fruits and vegetables, and helps regulate hormone balance, boost brain function, and improve immunity. L-theanine is found in green and white tea, and helps you fall asleep and remain asleep. It can elevate your levels of GABA, dopamine, and serotonin. In addition to protecting your cell membranes, myo-inositol increases chemical messengers in your brain, helps improve mood, and reduces the frequency and severity of mood-related symptoms.

Serotonin for Brain Repair and Higher-Brain Function

When serotonin is scarce, the hippocampus is unable to repair from the ongoing assault from cortisol. Learning stops. Your fluid intelligence—your ability to reason, think flexibly, and solve new problems—declines rapidly. You begin to depend on the way things used to be, unable to adapt to a dynamically changing world. Your thinking becomes fossilized regardless of your age.

For some still-unknown reasons, nature decided to make the hippocampus rich in receptors for cortisol and easily damaged by trauma. But nature also decided to give us serotonin to help us repair this learning center of the brain. Serotonin induces neurogenesis, the creation of new neurons to repair the brain.

Serotonin has a similar chemical signature to the potent psychedelic ingredient in ayahuasca, the brew prepared by the Amazonian healers that I had a chance to work with many years before it became popular with Westerners. The active ingredient in ayahuasca, DMT, has a strong affinity for the serotonin receptors in the brain.

The resemblance between serotonin and DMT begs the question: Why do our brains have receptors for such a powerful consciousness-altering substance? Receptors function like a lock-and-key mechanism, where a specific key is required to open a particular lock. A molecule like DMT (the key) connects exclusively with a specific receptor (the lock). Could it be that nature intended for us to discover mind-expanding brews to help the brain evolve higher-order circuitry, create new technologies, and experience a greater reality? Why do our brains naturally produce psychedelics, readily converting serotonin into DMT and other "spirit molecules" like mescaline, psilocybin, and LSD?

Our neocortex craves the spirit molecules. If your brain is missing an upgrade and you cannot manufacture your own, you might find yourself searching for psychedelics at weekend raves. You might even try microdosing magic mushrooms—heeding your brain's craving for an experience of Oneness. But the Grow a New Brain program offers more than just a weekend's adventure that might quickly be forgotten. It primes your brain to manufacture your own bliss molecules daily and the neural networks that allow you to experience Oneness and profound intuitive insight.

The ancient Greeks called it gnosis.

When your higher brain recovers the helm from your M-brain, and shuts down the production of stress hormones, the toxic web of modern life peels off to reveal your profound and abiding communion with nature. The ancients (and today's Amazon peoples) know that the forest and the ocean can teach you everything you need to know.

SKY GAZING

Sky gazing is a practice of certain monks in Tibet, and has tremendous health benefits. Not only do you get the good vitamin D your body needs but the photons from morning light also set the circadian rhythms in your brain. With this exercise, you welcome the light of the sun at dawn and connect through your breath with nature around you. Even if you live in a busy city with no parks, you can imagine yourself in a forest or in the Amazon.

Practice sky gazing in the early morning. Sit in a comfortable chair with your hands resting gently on your lap, eyes open, gazing straight ahead into the horizon. Take deep, gentle breaths. As you follow your breathing, witness everything that surfaces in your awareness as if it were a cloud in the sky that appears and disappears of its own accord. Notice when your mind wanders off, and coax it back gently to focus on your breath as you enjoy the morning sky. Just as clouds come and go, thoughts come and go, and sensations come and go.

With practice, all of the busyness and worries of the mind dissolve and you witness every feeling and thought with a smile.

A Lesson in the Jungle

When I was a young anthropologist traveling through the Peruvian Amazon, I visited a renowned medicine woman, and after having lunch at her home, we left the village to go for a walk through the forest. We arrived at a clearing by the edge of the Ucayali River, and the old woman indicated for me to walk across the field and notice what happened to the songs of the birds when I entered the jungle on the other side.

I walked over the soft wild grass, and when I entered the jungle again, I could hear the singing of the birds, the loud cackle of the macaws, and the monkeys in the distance. After three steps, everything stopped. The jungle became still as if the animals were sensing the presence of a predator. Even I became concerned, thinking there may be a jaguar nearby.

The shaman then came up to me and said, "The animals know that you don't belong here. They know that you've been kicked out of the garden and that you don't belong in their forest!" Strangely, as she drew near me, I noticed that the creatures of the rainforest had all begun singing again.

I thought that surely, she was making fun of me, thinking that I'm just a city boy from California.

There were two Shipibo men at a bend in the river nearby, and they were roasting a boa on a spit—their late lunch. They were collecting the boa fat in a can, and I went up to them and asked if I could have some of the snake fat. I was convinced that the animals were simply smelling my deodorant and toothpaste, scents I might be able to disguise by smearing myself with the boa fat.

I stripped down to my shorts and started lathering the boa fat on my body. I was convinced that when I returned to the rainforest, the animals were going to smell just another snake slithering back into the jungle. I noticed that the men were looking at me strangely, so I explained, "It's okay. I'm an anthropologist."

When I finished smearing myself in boa fat, I thanked the men and walked back into the jungle. The first step was full of song and so was the second step. And the third step. But then, once again, the harmonious cacophony stopped, except for the buzzing of about 600 flies swarming around me.

A full decade had to pass before I was able to venture into the rainforest and feel it acknowledging me as a rightful citizen of its realm. No longer an exile from the garden, I had joined "all my relations" who communed with the river and conversed with the ancient trees, as our kind had done in the primordial fields of Eden. The birds continued singing around me. In that moment, I realized that in years past I *had* been a trespasser, an alien presence amid its mysteries even as I enjoyed a stroll through a wood or a park, engrossed in thoughts about work.

After a half-dozen ayahuasca sessions in the Amazon and the abundant serotonin in my brain, my hippocampus began to repair from the trauma I had experienced during childhood. My fight-or-flight system reset to deep calm and safety. The animals no longer smelled my fear, no longer sensed the adrenaline in my blood. I realized that the creatures of the rainforest had the same reaction to my fear that I had when I heard no sound in the rainforest: Where was the jaguar? Where was the predator that was scaring this poor man?

Years after that initial sojourn into the Amazon, I finally discovered that I was an integral part of the garden, an essential yet insignificant thread in the tapestry of life. I had achieved that elusive state of Oneness. (Notice the similarity between DMT and serotonin. The chemical formula for serotonin is $C_{10}H_{12}N_2O$. The formula for DMT is $C_{12}H_{16}N_2$.)

Nonetheless, the scientific intellect that I had cultivated throughout my doctoral work and my tenure in the neuroscience laboratory became like an itch I needed to scratch. It whispered to me that my newfound communion was the result of healing the trauma that once clung to me like a shroud. The rainforest had embraced me, which was comforting, but it fell short of the profound connection I sought—the unconditional embrace from Mother Earth herself that I so longed for.

Psychology and the Earth Mother, Pachamama

Meanwhile, back in the United Sates, my psychotherapist was telling me that I had to deal with my mommy issues. "Pachamama is not going to make up for your mother not breast-feeding you," he said to me. And for two years I dug into that never-ending dark hole of trying to heal the mother wound that we all carry. It wasn't until I decided to increase the levels of serotonin in my brain with L-tryptophan supplements in the morning and 5-HTP in the evening, which powered my brain to manufacture its own DMT, that I found deep healing. I had to repair my hippocampus. I had to kick-start my pineal gland to produce melatonin and the bliss molecules. Only then could I have an aha moment and discover a new map that included the scientific disciplines that I had learned. Remember: The hippocampus is where we create and store the maps of what we consider possible for ourselves and our lives.

The sign of my recovery lay in my newfound ability to commune with the plants and converse directly with the Earth Mother herself.

"You are talking to the trees?" my therapist asked.

"Yes," I said.

I wanted to be careful of the Western hubris of attributing my newfound sense of peace to brain chemistry only. Deep healing requires forgiveness, acceptance, and responding to your calling to bring peace and beauty to others and become a steward of nature, an Earthkeeper. The brain chemistry is an important step, but it is only a step. Ultimately, we have to make our way back to the Great Mother, and to the Garden.

Where We Get Serotonin and Its Precursor, Tryptophan

Our brains are starved for serotonin.

In the brain, a small amount of serotonin is produced by neurons in the *raphe* nuclei in the brain stem. This cluster of cells produces serotonin from tryptophan. We cannot manufacture tryptophan. We must obtain it from our diet. In the gut, serotonin is also produced from tryptophan but only when you have a diverse and vibrant gut flora to manufacture it.

The reason for our serotonin deficiency, aside from our gut flora being damaged by antibiotics, is that for the last century, farmers have been breeding crops for sweetness because we have so many sweet taste receptors in our mouth. We've been breeding plants for sugar content. Ancient farmers were doing the opposite. They were breeding for serotonin. If you compare a chickpea from 400 years ago to one today, you'll find that the older one contained twice the amount of tryptophan. Ancient diets were providing us with the precursors for the bliss molecules to not only repair the hippocampus but also manufacture our own endogenous DMT.

So how did the early Americans fare with a diet based primarily on corn (representing about 80 percent of the caloric intake of the Pueblo people in the United States)? Starting around 1500 B.C.E., the diet of the inhabitants of the American Southwest included limited meat consumption. The population excelled at raising turkeys (which are rich in tryptophan). Yet these birds were primarily bred for their feathers, which were used in ceremonies. It turns out that the corn cultivated by these early Americans was host to a mushroom called *Ustilago maydis*, also known as "corn smut"—which increases the protein (and tryptophan) level in corn from about 3 percent to close to 20 percent.[5]

When you can't get tryptophan from today's foods, the results might be worse than poor sleep from lack of melatonin and bad moods. Studies the Food and Agriculture Organization of the United Nations published in the 1970s suggest that diets containing large amounts of corn (read sugars) may lead to aggressive and violent behavior, suggesting there may be a dietary explanation (rather than a sociocultural one) for high rates of homicide in modern Latin American nations.[6] Take Ecuador, for example. For a long time, a peaceful country sitting on the equator (thus the name), Ecuador is today one of the most violent regions in the world. Starting in the early 2000s, criminal gangs and drug cartels have overrun the country.

Is corn, which turns into sugar as soon as it hits the gut, the culprit? The Caral culture in central Peru was a cradle of civilization in the Andes that developed contemporaneously with those in Mesopotamia, Egypt, India, and China and dates back to approximately 3000 B.C.E. One of the finest achievements of the Caral civilization was its urban centers. The inhabitants of Caral constructed monumental structures, including pyramids, plazas, and residential complexes, requiring advanced engineering and architectural skills.

The Caral civilization is unusual by its absence of warfare; there is no evidence to suggest that the Caral people engaged in military conflicts. This peaceful coexistence was likely facilitated by their economic practices, which were reliant on trade, agriculture, and fishing. The Caral people cultivated crops such as cotton, squash, and beans, and their diet was supplemented by fish and seafood, obtained from the nearby Pacific Ocean. Their diet did not include corn. And there are no indications of mass burials or decapitations or armaments or protective walls to ward off enemies in any of their cities or plazas. They seem to have been peace-loving peoples.

I believe that the meager amount of serotonin our broken gut is able to manufacture from our diet can't satisfy the demands of our modern brains. Gut serotonin gives priority to peristalsis, making sure we can digest our food and move out wastes. What little remains will travel to the brain if, and only if, we are eating power plants that allow the passage of serotonin from the gut into the bloodstream and into the vagus nerve. These include many of the products discussed in this book, including curcumin, omega-3s, *Rhodiola rosea*, and most green plants.

But what about the serotonin produced inside the brain? For tryptophan to enter the brain, where it can be used to make serotonin, it must be ferried across the blood-brain barrier by a carrier, a "trucking company" that also shuttles into the brain isoleucine, leucine, and valine. These three BCAAs, or branched-chain amino acids (so-called because their molecular structure has "branches"), are commonly found in red meat, milk, and eggs. The BCAAs compete with tryptophan to be transported into the brain. When you're consuming an excessive amount of these animal products, the "trucking company" favors the BCAAs, and tryptophan loses out. The more you reduce your consumption of animal proteins to the levels of our hunter-gatherer ancestors, the happier you will be—because tryptophan will have less competition from the BCAAs to shuttle into the brain. And this is especially important because tryptophan is one of the least abundant amino acids in our diet.

But why would nature give priority to the BCAAs over tryptophan? It's because these amino acids are necessary to build your brain inside the womb and throughout your life. And in past millennia we only ate animal products occasionally, much as people in the Blue Zones consume today. The BCAA help build muscle, which is why bodybuilders consume them in large quantities. But as you'll learn in Chapter 9: Make Use of Powerful Pathways for Brain Health, BCAAS are the prime drivers of a pathway called MTOR and, eventually, the growth of unwanted tumors. Bodybuilders who use one or more "muscle supplements" increase their risk for testicular cancer by 177 percent.[7] Fortunately, there's a way to get ample protein into your brain without increasing your risk for cancer: consuming plant proteins.

As you repair your hippocampus with serotonin, your pineal gland will produce melatonin to reset your biological clock and allow you to sleep restfully. And if your fight-or-flight system is not signaling that there's a five-alarm fire happening when really, you're just imagining a threat rather than actually in danger, you have a chance of switching on the pineal gland's production of the bliss molecule—DMT—that can help you understand what your life is about.

But in addition to getting sufficient tryptophan, which you can purchase online in powdered form as L-tryptophan, you need to be sure you get adequate 5-HTP.

The Role of 5-HTP in Creating Serotonin

The amino acid 5-HTP (HTP stands for hydroxytryptophan), like tryptophan, is an essential serotonin precursor. If you decide to try this supplement (made from the seeds of the African shrub *Griffonia simplicifolia*), start with 100 mg, as more can make you feel nauseous. While that can be uncomfortable, it is a sign that the 5-HTP is improving signaling from your gut-brain axis. I take

L-tryptophan some mornings (about 200 mg or half a teaspoonful), and I watch how my mood improves and my day becomes brighter. Both supplements can be easily ordered online. I recommend you do not use it more than two or three times a week, in small doses.

If your gut flora is healthy, if you have the building blocks for serotonin (namely, L-tryptophan and 5-HTP), you will improve your mood. Anxiety levels will go down, your hippocampus will repair, and you will be able to have a new experience of health and life.

But this is only the beginning.

You will be taking 5-HTP for 10 days as part of the Grow a New Brain protocol. Then, as you are resting and sleeping well, you can begin to explore the gift of gnosis!

The Payoffs of Sufficient Serotonin

The first benefit you will experience after your brain gets adequate serotonin is that you will change the set point of your fight-or-flight system. You will begin to see your life, your job, and your spouse with different eyes. Your sessions with your therapist will transform from complaining and griping sessions, like mine had become, into ones in which you discover opportunities to reimagine your childhood experiences and your relationships in a positive light. Your moods will no longer depend on good news or bad news. This will happen when you have repaired your hippocampus, which is where we keep the navigation charts with the dangers and opportunities we may find in our life journey. Remember that the hippocampus has spatial, map-making intelligence. London taxi drivers have larger hippocampi than most people because they learn a large catalog of spatial information to traverse the complex layout of London.[8]

In many cultures, girls and women face limited chances to hone their driving abilities, contributing to the myth that they are naturally less adept at navigation compared to men. This belief is largely due to societal stereotypes, even when their actual performance matches that of men. Interestingly, it is older men who are most prone to overestimating their navigational skills when they take up the sport of orienteering.

You can't heal from trauma if you don't have the brain chemistry to repair the hippocampus. Psychologists are often baffled when they have to acknowledge that the mind requires the brain chemistry to grow the awareness that may allow you to fathom the pain from your childhood (or other trauma) and to reach atonement and forgiveness. You can't achieve these simply with words or by an act of willpower. You can't feel peaceful if your brain is awash in stress hormones. Likewise, we need DMT, to understand our place in the world and the cosmos. And it is as if Mother Nature knew we would require serotonin, and thus made it abundant to all life on earth.

However, to produce the bliss molecule DMT you need to be able to methylate properly. Many of us have methylation difficulties because we have a variant of the MTHFR gene, which helps the body process folate. (Folate is the natural form of vitamin B_9 found in leafy green vegetables, citrus fruits, and beans.) I have this gene variant and need to supplement with folic acid and a B-vitamin complex. Gene variants are common, and there are many people in the world who have one or two variants of the MTHFR gene. Regardless, when you're using the Grow a New Brain program, you will be supporting the production of endogenous DMT with B vitamins.

In fact, combining B vitamins with omega-3s is a magic formula for increasing BDNF. The combination can enhance cognition in older individuals as demonstrated in the Oxford VITACOG trial,[9] where participants with high omega-3 levels experienced a 68 percent reduction in brain shrinkage when also treated with B vitamins. This helps explain the previous failures of near-sighted studies that focused solely on B vitamins or omega-3 fatty acids. It seems that the effectiveness of B vitamins is dependent on individuals having a good omega-3 fatty acid status, and vice versa.

The Garden—and the Gut

Cranking up the production of your own "spirit molecules" is essential for providing the gateways for us to make our way back to Eden, to our natural states.

But to do this we need to rewrite the story of the serpent.

A new way of looking at the story of our adventures in the Garden of Eden is by entertaining the thought that the serpent, which was coiled around the Tree of the Knowledge, was the tree's guardian. The serpent is a symbol of the goddess in ancient Mediterranean cultures, and of the awakening of consciousness and sexuality, and was tasked with bringing the fruit of wisdom to the woman so that "her eyes would be opened." This is what our endogenous DMT achieves. The spirit molecules open our eyes to a greater reality, what the ancients refer to as gnosis, to the Akashic Field, or the Implicit Order.

Today, we need the ability to create the neural networks in our higher brain to free ourselves from the original wound of shame, of being cast out and betrayed by our mother, Eve, and the habit of blaming the feminine (and women—in particular, our mothers) for our fate. Perhaps it can also help us make our way back to the garden, taste directly the fruit of wisdom, and stop the demeaning of wise women. Otherwise, we will remain in the shackles of the lower brain, keeping women and girls living in fear, shame, and scarcity.

You don't need to flood your brain with DMT to experience its benefits. Nano doses of DMT manufactured by the pineal gland will allow you to meditate and find a sense of communion with nature. And after you have managed to quiet your mind, you may be able to hear the voice of Spirit in the wind and speak with ancient trees to learn their wisdom. You will learn that Spirit has not stopped communicating with us, that we are the ones who have stopped listening.

Key Takeaways:

We explored the themes of sleep, your biological clock, and the importance of serotonin.

1. Resetting your sleep cycle by getting early morning sunshine or using a panel with blue LEDs to help set your biological clock and treat seasonal depression during shorter days of winter.

2. Lack of quality sleep harms the brain, as it shrinks by 20 percent while sleeping, allowing cerebral spinal fluid to flush away toxins.

3. How insufficient serotonin levels can lead to difficulty falling and staying asleep, as well as disrupted sleep cycles.

4. How the craving for spirit molecules by the highly developed neocortex might lead to using psychedelics, and how the Grow a New Brain program offers a different approach by priming the brain to produce the spirit molecules and install neural networks for profound intuitive insight and experiences of Oneness.

Chapter 9

MAKE USE OF POWERFUL PATHWAYS FOR BRAIN HEALTH

Our bodies have powerful pathways that play critical roles in delaying aging, the prevention of disease, and most importantly protecting our brains. We'll look at the mTOR, IGF1, and Nrf2 pathways, but first, I want you to understand the master controller of aging, which developed billions of years ago when the only forms of life on the planet were bacteria.

mTOR and Protein

When the earth was young, bacteria populated the waters and developed a kind of "radar" sensor to detect the presence of food. The law of life back then, like today, was eat or be eaten. When food (protein) was abundant, the bacteria feasted and went into a growth and reproduction mode. When the sensor detected little or no protein, they entered into hibernation, until the sensor sent the message, "Hey, I've found a terrific supply of bacteria you can eat." At this point, the bacteria switched back to growth and making offspring—and so it went, in a cycle of dormancy or reproduction based on the amount of food available. Modern humpback whales still follow a pattern of seasonal eating, feasting during six months of the year and fasting the other six months as they mate.

The protein sensor those early life-forms developed is called TOR, or *target of rapamycin*, and it's found in every microbe, animal, and plant. This sensor was only recently discovered and is named after the drug rapamycin. In mammals, we call TOR the mammalian target of rapamycin, or "MTOR." As winter approaches and food becomes scarce, a brown bear's MTOR system signals them to find a cave to curl up in until spring arrives. Hibernation is an example of MTOR switching on the systems for survival during times of food scarcity. In Europe during World War II, when starvation posed a very real threat, MTOR halted women's fertility. They were unable to conceive despite remaining sexually active. Their bodies recognized that this was not a good time to be making babies, which would deplete the mother of hard-to-obtain nutrients and endanger her life. Thus, MTOR switched women's bodies to survival and repair mode.

Similarly, MTOR ensures the survival of future generations during times of famine. Regulating MTOR to induce our body to bring us into repair and regeneration is the secret to growing a new body and brain. We can achieve this through the Grow a New Brain protocol, which supplies first-rate neuro-nutrients to help repair and rebuild your brain.

How Many Years Are We Designed to Live?

When older animals die, the next generation can flourish and the species evolves, with new genetic variations appearing in the offspring. Nature doesn't want elderly males intent on spreading their own seed to live forever, blocking the potential of genetic novelty created by a variety of pairings between males and females. Nature also isn't particularly keen on grandmothers. Elderly members of the species are picked off by predators or afflicted by disease caused by the breakdown of their free-radical scavenging systems. Curiously, only humans, whales, and dolphins have the luxury of having, and perhaps becoming, grandmothers. Females of other species can't entertain the possibility of healthy senior years. For them, the MTOR program runs full speed during youth and then dooms them when reproduction—the primary agenda of biology— is no longer feasible. In the wild, when animals can't make babies any longer, they die. That's not the destiny you or I want.

We humans—like dolphins and whales—are lucky in that we don't have a premature death sentence encoded in our DNA, which all other species have. The average life expectancy of a woman in the United States is 79 years. That is more or less four decades after her childbearing years. There's no genetic design for us to die early from natural causes. In other words, these three species are taking part in an amazing biological experiment in longevity.

Today we know how to switch off the genes for age-related disease, and switch on the ones for a long, healthy life. We know how to downregulate MTOR to slow down aging without needing to starve. But we have to do several things, including watching our animal protein intake, because the MTOR clock is still ticking inside every one of us, monitoring our consumption of animal foods.

Protein, MTOR, and the Risk of an Overactive Pathway

Protein is important. Before the age of 20, you need plenty of dietary protein to grow a strong body and brain. Nature wants you to buff up and get desirable and sexy to ensure the survival of the species. In your later years, you also need additional protein to prevent muscle wasting. Yet in the 60 years between the age of 20 and 80, excess animal protein will trigger premature aging. The average American is said to ingest 274 pounds of beef per year, not including seafood and fish.[1] In contrast, people in the Blue Zones (Icaria, Greece, and Okinawa, Japan, among others), the longest-lived people on earth, consume on average very small portions of meat: two ounces four to five times per month. This is like two bites of meat per week!

With plant-based protein in your diet, the MTOR pathway is humming quietly. Cells are born, grow, divide, and die in an organic rhythm, recycling their content during autophagy. You get rid of the old and broken-down mitochondria and recycle 95 percent or more of their protein, greatly diminishing the need for dietary intake of animal products. When you find yourself craving animal protein (like a steak), it is often a sign that you are not recycling properly, autophagy is not working, and toxins are building up in your system, causing accelerated aging.

When MTOR is activated, it's like stepping on the accelerator of a car. Autophagy and recycling end. Cells grow and divide more quickly and can lead to uncontrolled proliferation of unwanted cells. You can think of overactivated MTOR and faster cell growth like an unchecked wildfire: It starts out small and containable, but if not taken care of, it spreads, and rapidly. The result is serious damage to the environment—in this case, the environment is your body. And unlike a forest that will replenish itself over time, your body won't be able to recover easily. We call this accelerated aging and decrepitude—or early onset dementia and cognitive decline. And we think it is natural and normal, but it is not. If your MTOR pathway is overly active because you're consuming excessive quantities of animal products, you have a good chance of ending up in poor health, on multiple medications, and on the fast track to aging.

To prevent these outcomes, you want to quiet the MTOR pathway.

A WONDER DRUG THAT DOWNREGULATES mTOR

In the year 1972, a discovery was made on Easter Island, or as its inhabitants call it, Rapa Nui. The peoples of this remote island in the Pacific Ocean crafted colossal stone statues of human figures with oversized heads between the 13th and 16th centuries. At the base of these statues, a fungus destined to change the course of medicine was thriving.

The drug rapamycin, made from the fungus discovered at the foot of the Moai, can suppress the body's immune response, important for individuals undergoing organ transplantation, as it prevents rejection by the recipient's own immune system. Rapamycin offered a renewed lease on life for many.

Rapamycin would eventually reveal a surprising side effect. Patients on this medication showed reduced rates of heart disease, cancer, and dementia in comparison with the general population and with those using other immunosuppressants. This discovery sparked a huge interest among longevity researchers, as rapamycin also had an excellent safety profile and had already been in use for decades.

Rapamycin exerts its magic by downregulating the activity of MTOR. It has a specific target called TORC1 (target of rapamycin complex 1), responsible for growth and the speed of human aging. Rapamycin tricks the body into believing it is going into starvation. In response, the body shifts from growth (and reproduction) to repair and regeneration, slowing the aging clock and the diseases that accompany aging.

Many physicians have incorporated rapamycin into their personal regimens, but it's difficult to find a doctor who will prescribe it even though the pills cost less than $1 per day—as its off-label use is not covered by insurance. Fortunately, it's possible to downregulate MTOR activity through dietary and lifestyle modifications. These allow you to achieve similar health benefits.

I personally take rapamycin as part of my prevention protocol; 5 mg once a week for seven weeks, then six weeks off.

Note that MTOR activation is not inherently bad; it plays an important role in protein synthesis and growth, especially during childhood. However, excessive or chronic activation of MTOR will accelerate the aging clock. In a balanced plant-based diet, the effects on MTOR are moderated and will not have the same deleterious effect as a diet heavily reliant on bacon and hamburgers.

Ways to Downregulate MTOR

To downregulate your MTOR during the 10-day Grow a New Brain program, start by significantly reducing or even eliminating from your diet sugar and animal products—especially meat, dairy, and eggs. Replace these products with plant-based food sources that are less likely to activate MTOR (you may eat small amounts of fish).[2] Consume sugars only in the form of berries, which have phytonutrients you'll need, and restrict your food intake to a six- to eight-hour window.

As you learned, meat, dairy, and eggs contain high amounts of leucine, isoleucine, and valine, known as BCAAs (branched-chain amino acids). Excessive BCAAs will up-regulate MTOR, which we don't want. In fact, MTOR radar picks up only the three BCAAs and no other protein forms. Sugar also upregulates MTOR, and in addition, it feeds *Candida* in your gut, disturbing the balance of your microbiome.

Eating during a 6-hour window and fasting the other 18 hours is my favorite method for downregulating MTOR. Biogerontologist Valter Longo at the University of Southern California shares the benefits of this practice. His studies have demonstrated that when subjected to time-restricted eating, laboratory animals not only experience an extension in their life span but are also less prone to developing disease as they grow older.

By engaging in time-restricted eating, you downregulate MTOR, paving the way for potential health benefits akin to those observed in longevity studies. For example, I will eat an early dinner at 6 P.M. and then not eat anything until noon the following day. The power of these few hours of fasting to modulate pathways for health high-lights the ability of lifestyle choices to impact our longevity.

DR. ALBERTO'S DIET

I eat a primarily plant-based ketogenic diet, which means that I am burning fats for brain fuel. My favorite sources of fats: avocado, olive oil, olives, almonds, walnuts, chia, chocolate, tahini, MCT, coconut oil, and fatty fish.

Every day I plan on a combination of cooked vegetables and soups that include seaweeds.

- Nonstarchy vegetables: spinach, broccoli, mushrooms, kale, cauliflower, zucchini, and bell peppers roasted in the oven
- Healthy fats: olive oil (sprinkled on everything!), coconut oil, avocados, and MCT oil
- Nuts: almonds, walnuts, cashews, macadamia nuts, and pistachios, which I snack on during the day
- Seeds: chia, hemp, flax, and pumpkin seeds
- Nut butters: almond, pecan, and hazelnut butter, which I make at home on a blender

- Other protein: tofu, tempeh, spirulina, and natto
- Low-carb fruits: wild blueberries, lemons, strawberries, and blackberries
- Herbs and seasonings: basil, paprika, pepper, turmeric, salt, oregano, rosemary, thyme, and chile peppers

These are phytochemical-rich foods. At mealtime, plant foods will dominate my plate! Yet most of my actual calories will come from fats like olive oil and avocados. In addition, I have a big helping of broccoli sprouts on my salad four days per week.

One benefit to not eating late in the evening and delaying your breakfast in the morning is that you'll cue your brain to go into ketosis and run on fats rather than sugars. Restricting your window for eating to six to eight hours will help you maintain ketosis. That in turn will trigger autophagy and the recycling of cellular wastes. Your MTOR system will signal for you to go into repair and regeneration.

During ketosis, the ketones produced from our own fat stores include β-hydroxybutyrate (BHB), an especially excellent fuel for the brain that will activate your frontal lobes—your God brain. That's because BHB is jet fuel for mitochondria, many times as powerful as sugars.

During the 10-day Grow a New Brain program, you will get the protein your body needs from autophagy, so you can regenerate the brain. You'll detoxify. And you will avoid ending up in dementia land.

If you're worried about getting enough protein, I have good news. Eliminating sugar and taking quality probiotics means you will eradicate the unwanted yeast and bacteria in your gut, allowing the good ones to colonize. As you repair your microbiome, you will be able to better extract amino acids from the plant-based foods you eat, giving you plenty of protein. Plant-based proteins are less easily digested than animal proteins, because they are tightly bound in plant cell walls. So if you feel you are not getting sufficient protein from your plant-based diet, it could be a sign that your gut microbiome is in need of an upgrade.

The Mayo Clinic website states: "The recommended dietary allowance to prevent deficiency for an average sedentary adult is 0.8 grams per kilogram of body weight. For example, a person who weighs 165 pounds, or 75 kilograms, should consume 60 grams of protein per day."[3] As much as I respect the Mayo Clinic, I am convinced that if our autophagy is functioning properly, we only need half of this amount, and we do not have to get them in a single sitting. We all have enough protein in our cellular "recycling bins" to last us for several weeks! And remember that excess protein is stored as fat! What's important is to be sure your body is burning fat for fuel so you can kick-start autophagy—recycling the tremendous storehouse of proteins you have available in every cell. You can build new cells using 95 percent of the recycled protein. If you are not recycling, you are accumulating cellular waste and senescent cells. (You'll learn about the latter in Chapter 10: Arm Yourself for the Zombie Invasion: Eliminating Senescent Cells with Plant Medicines.)

AUTOPHAGY AND THE NEED FOR OLD AND DAMAGED CELLS TO DIE

Autophagy is a process where cells break down and recycle their own components. The term *autophagy* comes from the Greek words *auto*, meaning "self," and *phagy*, meaning "eating." Remember that every cell and tissue in your body is constantly growing and breaking down, continually renewing itself. This is the turnover rate of proteins, and the turnover rate of your brain is three times as fast as your muscles, including your heart! Autophagy helps cells recycle aging mitochondria, misfolded proteins, and eliminate pathogens. It protects cells under stress, such as during starvation. By breaking down old components, autophagy provides new cells with necessary building blocks. (Here is how it works: It begins with the formation of a small, fluid-filled bladder called an autophagosome, that swallows damaged cellular components and then fuses with a lysosome, a sphere containing enzymes for breaking down proteins. The resulting amino acids are used by the cell for building proteins to make muscle and blood and many of the 200 different kinds of cells in the body.)

When autophagy is not working properly because you are consuming too much animal products or sugar, damaged cells accumulate and accelerate aging.

The IGF-1 Pathway, Activated by Sugar

IGF-1 (insulin-like growth factor 1) works with growth hormones to promote healthy growth of bone and tissue during childhood and helps in tissue repair throughout your life. But when you are older, a high level of IGF-1 is deadly, as we do not need to grow any new fingers or toes, and shortens your life span by activating MTOR.

Ordinary blood tests measure your IGF-1 levels, and testing is a good way to sense whether your body is on a roller coaster toward dementia. Since IGF-1 levels vary for everyone, there is only a personal, individual, ideal level, and I prefer being toward the lower end of the scale but not so low that I am not repairing tissue! As you reduce your sugar consumption, notice how your IGF-1 level drops. High-protein diets have also been linked to increased IGF-1, so again watch your animal protein intake.

Longevity

Despite the many different life spans observed in mammals, smaller species generally tend to have "faster" life histories. The hormone IGF-1 seems to regulate life span. Elevated IGF-1 levels are linked to faster life histories, with rapid growth and reproduction but dying young. For example, the Indian elephant can live up to 65 years, and has a lower level of IGF-1 (by body weight) than the house mouse with a high IGF-1 and that lives on average around 2 years.

Zoologists Eli Swanson and Ben Dantzer studied 41 mammalian species and found that high IGF-1 levels correspond to shortened life span.[4] Their findings suggest that IGF-1s is a regulator of longevity conserved across all mammals. What does this mean for us humans? Given that sugar and excess protein increase your levels of IGF-1, which then turns up MTOR, we may want to consider maintaining our individual IGF-1 levels toward the lower area of the normal spectrum, lest we unnecessarily shorten our life spans. I like to keep my IGF-1 levels around 120, which most doctors consider to be on the low side.

The takeaway so far in this chapter is that both animal protein and refined sugar will make you grow older faster, and thus bring on the diseases associated with aging. Stay with me, because we are going to go a little deeper into biology . . .

The Nrf2 Pathway: The "Shaman's Pathway"

Amazonian dwellers discovered that certain plants allowed them to remain in exceptional health. These plants did not treat diseases; they *prevented* them. Today, we know these as adaptogens that help the body respond to stress and create overall health.

Adaptogens have been employed for thousands of years in traditional folk medicine. These plants and mushrooms help your body deal with stress, anxiety, and fatigue, and return to health. They have a broad, nonspecific beneficial effect on the body's ability to adapt. They help you respond to stressors. Ashwagandha, bacopa, and rhodiola are three adaptogens we will use in our recipes for beverages later in the book. Some of my favorite adaptogens are mushrooms, including reishi, lion's mane, turkey tail, and cordyceps.

BRAIN MUSHROOMS

Reishi (*Ganoderma lucidum*), called the "mushroom of immortality," is revered in traditional Asian medicine for its health-enhancing properties. Thought to boost immune response, reishi mushrooms help the body fend off pathogens. Reishi reduces stress and promotes mental clarity and relaxation. Its anti-inflammatory and antioxidant properties can reduce the risk of chronic diseases and support heart health by balancing blood pressure and cholesterol levels. Reishi is known for improving sleep quality and combating fatigue, making it a stellar performer for enhancing physical health and well-being. Reishi upregulates BDNF and balances the levels of neurotransmitters in the brain, playing a key role in regulating your mood.

Lion's mane (*Hericium erinaceus*) is a nootropic fungus known for benefits to brain health and cognitive function. It is rich in molecules that stimulate the production of BDNF and nerve growth factor (NGF), both crucial for the survival of neurons. This mushroom can enhance cognitive functions, including memory, attention, and creativity, and may protect against the development of neurodegenerative diseases. Its anti-inflammatory properties support gut health and the immune system. It is also an antioxidant, reducing oxidative stress and inflammation.

Turkey tail (*Trametes versicolor*) has a fan-shaped, multicolored appearance, hence the name. It is packed with polysaccharides, which make it a powerful immunomodulator, which means it can help regulate the immune system, enhancing the activity of natural killer cells in response to pathogens. This mushroom has been extensively studied and used in conjunction with cancer therapy in Asia. Additionally, turkey tail has a high antioxidant content, reducing oxidative stress and inflammation and lowering the risk of chronic diseases. It's a prebiotic, promoting the growth of beneficial gut bacteria, essential for maintaining a healthy digestive system.

Cordyceps (*Cordyceps sinensis* and *militaris*) boosts energy and endurance and contain cordycepin, a compound that enhances the body's production of energy at a cellular level. Cordyceps is a favorite among athletes seeking improved performance and reduced fatigue. Additionally, cordyceps has been linked to improved respiratory health, with benefits for asthma and bronchitis sufferers due to its anti-inflammatory properties. It also helps maintain healthy cholesterol levels and improve circulation. Cordyceps strengthens the immune system by enhancing the activity of natural killer cells and regulating blood sugar levels.

In Tibetan folklore, cordyceps was discovered by yak herders who noticed that their animals became more energetic and lively after consuming the fungus. It was once so highly prized that it was exclusively reserved for the emperors of China.

The Nrf2

Nuclear factor erythroid 2-related factor 2 (I can't pronounce it either . . .) is the master regulator of cellular defenses.

Nrf2 is a protein that rests quietly on the cell's membrane—but when it is activated by broccoli sprouts you will grow in your kitchen laboratory, it penetrates into the nucleus of the cell to launch a cascade of protective detoxification genes. Nrf2 activates Quinone Reductase (NQ01), which has been described as a "quintessential cytoprotective (cell protective) enzyme."[5] Nrf2 was discovered in 2002 by Shyam Biswal, a scientist at the Johns Hopkins School of Medicine. He and his team found that Nrf2 controls the rate at which information is copied from DNA. You can think of Nrf2 as being like a conductor leading an orchestra, maintaining the overall harmony while occasionally highlighting the violins or the drums. In this case, the "violins" are the antioxidants like glutathione and SOD, which neutralize free radicals. Nrf2, as Biswal explained, is the master regulator of detoxification in the body.

Biswal and his team discovered that the detoxification system loses resilience around age 35 when we are past our child-bearing years. Yet the Nrf2 protein, once it enters the nucleus and has access to our DNA, can turn these systems back on again, restoring immunity and restarting our production of glutathione and SOD. The Nrf2 activators you will learn to use in the Grow a New Brain program will return your antioxidant production to the levels you had when you were in your 20s!

While we have genes that protect against cellular damage, it's Nrf2 that gets them to do their job—cuing the drum section to begin to play, so to speak. Until recently, the power of Nrf2 has been attributed to its antioxidant properties, but Nrf2 has the ability to influence large banks of other genes as well. Three hours after Nrf2 has been activated by broccoli sprouts, more than 1725 genes that create health will have been switched on. And in 12 hours, nearly 4,000 protective genes will have been switched on in total—and the Nrf2 pathway will remain active for more than 24 hours.[6]

The Nrf2 will restore the levels of antioxidants, drug metabolizing enzymes, heat shock proteins, NAD enzymes, growth factors, and heavy metal–binding proteins, which decline precipitously around the age of 35 years.

The rescue remedy of the body? Nrf2.

However, even if you have sufficient Nrf2 outside the membranes of your cells in standby mode, it might not do its job. You must activate the Nrf2.

Activating the Nrf2 Pathway

Millennia ago, Amazon peoples discovered the plants that held the secrets to preventing disease. Today we know that they are Nrf2 activators.

Plants have defense systems against predators that threaten their survival. For example, a bug chewing on the leaves or stem of a broccoli sprout will activate the plant's immune system, and trigger the release of defensive chemicals in much the same way that our own bodies mount an immune response when we are bitten by a mosquito. The beauty of some chemicals that protect plants is that they are also astonishingly effective for humans for preventing disease—by activating our Nrf2 pathway. The most stellar are these:

Sulforaphane: When insects chew on young broccoli shoots, a compound known as sulforaphane is released, a powerful chemical that keeps bugs at bay and repairs damage to young shoots.

Sulforaphane is the most potent Nrf2 activator we know as well as the most bioavailable (more easily absorbed by the body). Some plants that are particularly rich in sulforaphane include kale, cabbage, and Brussels sprouts, but by far, the best source for it is broccoli—and better yet, broccoli sprouts that germinate from seeds in your kitchen!

You cannot buy sulforaphane supplements. The best you can do is to purchase glucoraphanin, which your body can turn into sulforaphane—but only if you have a natural supply of the enzyme myrosinase in your gut. If your gut is compromised from antibiotic use and a poor diet, the alchemy will not happen; the glucoraphanin will go right through you unused. That's why it's a good idea to grow your own broccoli sprouts in your kitchen laboratory. And you'll want to chew them well to release sulforaphane *in your mouth*—as if you were a rabbit munching on sprouts in the wild. Crush the sprouts by chopping, blending, or chewing them; then, the magic occurs.

You will notice results as your Nrf2 system kicks into action, increasing antioxidant production and regenerating tissues, including the wrinkles on your face. It will also reduce the ability of deviant cells to multiply, slowing tumor growth and keeping tumors from migrating to other parts of the body. In fact, if a man eats just three servings of broccoli a week (which is much less powerful than the sprouts), he cuts his risk of prostate cancer by a whopping 60 percent![7]

In addition, sulforaphane helps build bone density and protect against osteoporosis.[8] And your broccoli sprouts provide another excellent benefit: They activate the detoxifying genes that eliminate the heavy metals arsenic and lead in your body. In Chapter 11, you'll learn how to grow your own broccoli sprouts so you can get real sulforaphane into your body and brain.

Pterostilbene (pronounced tero-STILL-bean) is a phytonutrient (*phyto* means plant) found in blueberries and also grapes, grape leaves, and almonds. Pterostilbene is related to another Nrf2 activator, resveratrol, which is also found in fruits, but it's more bioavailable. This nutrient has gained attention for its health benefits, which include being a potent anti-inflammatory that supports cognitive function. Pterostilbene will inhibit the growth of cancer cells in vitro and induce apoptosis in many types of cancer; it will also activate the sirtuin proteins, particularly sirtuin 1, which promotes increased life span and improved metabolic health.

Coffee, which contains pyrocatechol, is a potent Nrf2 activator.[9] Best to think of coffee as a potent drug than a recreational drink. I began drinking coffee on the advice of a doctor friend many years ago. He told me about research that shows coffee drinkers have lower rates of liver cancer than non-coffee drinkers, but he couldn't tell me why. The science now shows that if you drink two or more cups of coffee a day, you reduce your risk for liver cancer and fibrosis by nearly 45 percent![10] I believe that it's because Nrf2 activation provides protection from cancers.

We need the power plants that are rich in Nrf2 activators. These plants hold the secret keys to health and longevity.

The Power Plants

The keys to growing a new body and upgrading your brain are the plants rich in Nrf2 activators. I make sure to take a variety of them during the week, every week of the year, but not during the 10-day Grow a New Brain protocol, when you will use nutritional supplements and not plants like the ones below. And while you can order most of these in capsule form, I prefer to buy the dried and powdered plants (you can order them easily online) and mix them into beverages in my kitchen laboratory. Whenever possible, I like to mix the plant extract—like curcumin—with the whole plant—turmeric—that has many molecules and pathways that work synergistically. Top plant-based adaptogens that are rich Nrf2 activators include:

Moringa (*Moringa oleifera*) is sometimes called the tree of life. It grows in India and triggers glutathione production inside every cell in the body, including the brain. It may have properties like sulforaphane, as it has a similar molecular structure, and is a potent antioxidant. Moringa leaves, which I like to buy in powder form, taste like spinach. You can use it in smoothies and soups. Check out the Matcha Energy Tonic recipe in the Appendix.

Curcumin/turmeric (*Curcuma longa*): Curcumin is the active ingredient in the Indian spice turmeric. It is a flowering plant of the ginger family used in curries. It continues gaining attention as a potent senolytic agent and activates genes for detoxification. Curcumin has also been shown in animal studies to counteract damage caused by radiation and chemotherapy as well as to restore kidney function and increase the life span of laboratory animals. I prepare a "golden milk" every evening mixing ¼ teaspoon curcumin powder plus a dash of turmeric (the whole plant, which works synergistically with the curcumin), mixing with warm almond milk, honey, and a dash of black pepper.

Green tea has more antioxidants and polyphenols than any other tea. It is rich in epigallocatechin-3-gallate (EGCG), which has been shown to be protective against lung, prostrate, skin, and breast cancer. One beneficial side effect of green tea is that it can help reduce body weight and fat mass.

Bacopa (*Bacopa monnieri*) has been employed in traditional folk remedies for longevity and cognitive enhancement. Considered a nootropic, bacopa is used in Ayurvedic medicine to improve cognitive function and memory, relieve stress and anxiety, and enhance mood. It grows in marshy areas on several continents, including Asia and South America, and is a calming cognitive enhancer. Bacopa has antidepressant and anxiolytic effects, reducing cortisol secretion and restoring the dopamine and serotonin depleted during chronic stress.

Mucuna (*Mucuna pruriens* or velvet bean) shines for its high content of L-DOPA, the precursor to dopamine. The surface of the bean is sticky because of a high concentration of serotonin. Adding mucuna to your tonics and smoothies will reduce the symptoms of Parkinson's disease as effectively as pharmaceutical medications, and early research shows that it may have all-around neuroprotective properties. In Ayurvedic medicine, it is used as an aphrodisiac, as a treatment for nervous system disorders, and even as an antidote to snake venom. Mucuna should not be used in conjunction with medications containing L-DOPA, which could produce excessively high dopamine levels.

Ashwagandha (*Withania somnifera*), a plant found in Asia and Africa, relieves stress and anxiety and sharpens focus and memory. It is known as the king of Ayurvedic herbs and boosts testosterone in men, increasing sperm quality and motility. It also increases focus and memory in both men and women.[11] Ashwagandha shines as an anxiolytic (antianxiety) and stress-relieving supplement. It improves sleep quality in people with and without insomnia.

Rhodiola (*Rhodiola rosea*) is an herb known for its ability to help the body resist physical, chemical, and biological stress. It is native to the cold regions of Europe and Asia, and its root is used in herbal medicine to enhance mental and physical endurance, reduce fatigue, and improve stress resilience. It grows readily in the wild Artic regions of northern Europe and central Asia. The Vikings ingested rhodiola to boost their endurance and strength, while in Siberia, people drank rhodiola tea in hopes it would help them live longer. The mechanism of action of rhodiola is still poorly understood.

Maca (*Lepidium meyenii*) is a plant native to the Andes Mountains of Peru and Bolivia, and is known as Peruvian ginseng. It has been used by Andean peoples for more than 2,000 years. The maca plant is rich in essential vitamins and minerals and highly regarded for its ability to enhance energy and stamina. Its benefits include increased libido and fertility in both men and women and helping the body better manage stress and balance hormone levels. Maca's nutrients support immune function, bone health, and cognitive function, reducing the risk of chronic diseases.

Gotu Kola (*Centella asiatica*) is a perennial plant that has been used for centuries in traditional Chinese, Ayurvedic, and African medicine. Its health benefits are attributed largely to saponins, flavonoids, and other phytochemicals. Gotu kola is renowned for its ability to enhance cognitive function. It improves memory and cognitive performance, boosting brain health and protecting against cognitive decline.

Cacao (*Theobroma cacao*): The name comes from the Greek "food of the gods." Native to Central and South America, cacao has been used ceremonially for generations. Cacao improves age-related neuronal dysfunction and neutralizes the impact of oxidative stress in the brain. My wife, Marcela, holds cacao ceremonies where we not only get the benefits of neuronal protection but also enjoy being in a sacred space. Cocoa extract and/or dark chocolate is associated with increased blood flow, and high levels of epicatechin will increase the production of nitric oxide as well as protect mitochondria.[12]

There are many other phytonutrient-rich plants that the Amazon peoples work with that are not available to us in the West. And when we work with power plants we have to be aware of the hormetic effect, that can turn nectar into poison.

Hormesis, and a Good Level of Biological Stress on the Body

The word *hormesis* is derived from the Greek word *hormáō* (ὁρμάω), which means "to set in motion" or "to urge on." Hormesis refers to when low doses of a potentially harmful substance can induce a positive response in an organism while higher doses may be toxic.

For example, low doses of sulforaphane can trigger the production of detoxifying enzymes and improve cellular defense systems. This is because your body identifies this compound as a possible toxin. Your cells react with a massive production of antioxidants (glutathione and SOD) to protect you against this perceived threat.

Because hormesis is dose dependent, small amounts of Nrf2 activators like sulforaphane in broccoli sprouts eaten four days a week, or drinking two or three cups of coffee no more than five days a week, have tremendously beneficial effects. But if you consume broccoli sprouts or drink coffee daily, the effect is negated, and you shut down the detoxification systems you want to activate, even as you still receive the full nutritional benefit! Everything, even water and oxygen, in excessive amounts, can be toxic. As Paracelsus, the 16th-century Swiss-German alchemist and physician, wrote, "All things are poison, and nothing is without poison; the dosage alone makes it so a thing is not a poison."[13]

The key to hormesis is cycling. I've modified my coffee intake to a cup or two every day for five days, then I'll skip it for a couple of days—switching over to green or black tea—before enjoying it again. Similarly, you want to eat your broccoli sprouts for four days, foregoing them for the next three and then repeating the cycle. Cycling with sulforaphane helps protect you from disease,[14] but you want to be sure you don't overdo your intake, or you'll shut down the very beneficial effects and get only the nutritional value. Remember, the hormetic healing effects require cycling, while the nutritional benefits do not.

Key Takeaways:

We explored the master regulators of longevity and the power plants that optimize brain performance.

1. The MTOR pathway, protein intake, and the effects of time-restricted eating on longevity and brain health.

2. The MTOR pathway is a critical factor in regulating aging, reproduction, and survival across different species. It plays a role in controlling growth and reproduction in response to food availability, and how regulating MTOR signaling could lead to benefits in overall health and longevity.

3. How MTOR can switch on systems for survival and maintenance during times of food scarcity, as seen in hibernation and historical instances of famine.

4. How the source and amount of dietary protein is a significant factor in MTOR regulation and aging. The cautions against excess animal protein and how it can trigger premature aging.

5. Time-Restricted Eating: A powerful method for downregulating MTOR and promoting longevity and brain health. The practice of fasting for extended periods and eating within a compressed window is associated with extending life span and reducing the risk of age-related diseases.

6. How time-restricted eating can lead to entering a state of ketosis, triggering autophagy and promoting the elimination of cellular wastes as part of the body's regeneration and repair processes.

Chapter 10

ARM YOURSELF FOR THE ZOMBIE INVASION

Eliminating Senescent Cells with Plant Medicines

Dozens of biotech companies are hoping to discover new drugs that will reverse aging, repair damaged organs, and rejuvenate wrinkled skin. They promise breakthroughs we'll see in the next decades, even ones that may allow us to live upward of 120 years! But unless you eat wisely and upgrade your brain and biology, you may not live long enough to take advantage of the discoveries that may permit longevity escape velocity, that is, adding more than one year of healthy life for every year you live.

It's hard to improve on biology, and biotech scientists are up against a 500-million-year R & D program designed by nature. Yet there is very exciting science in the works today.

I am intrigued by the Yamanaka factors. These four factors (formally known as Oct3/4, Sox2, Klf4, and c-Myc) are responsible for directing which genes turn on and off during embryonic development: some become liver cells, others become brain cells or skin cells, and so on. Introduce these four factors into mature cells and you can reprogram them into becoming pluripotent stem cells (which can differentiate into any type of cell in the body). Shinya Yamanaka, after whom these factors are named, received the Nobel Prize in Medicine in 2012 for the discovery that mature cells can be reprogrammed in this way. Biotech visionaries are inviting us to imagine a near future where you no longer must wait in line for a heart transplant or hip replacement but could grow whatever organ you need from your own cells, avoiding any danger of rejection!

We already have natural solutions to aging created by nature and discovered by Indigenous peoples. Suffice to say that the sages in Asia, Europe, and the Americas were consummate observers of the natural world and identified the plants and fungi that prevent disease and the remedies that keep you youthful into old age. Since time immemorial, power plants have been used for staving off the ravages of aging. The Chinese ruler known as the Yellow Emperor, who died in 2599 B.C.E. at the age of 110 years, wrote, "The Saint treats those ill-to-be rather than those being ill and cares for those in normality rather than those in chaos. Drug a disease after it's developed, or quench a chaos after it's evident—it's the same as digging a well when thirsty . . ."[1]

I prefer to focus on the amazing power of plants and fungi to promote resilience and lifelong health. Fortunately, nature gave us an abundance of plant medicines that can keep our body and brain healthy so we can enjoy the benefits of rejuvenation—biological tonics that cannot be owned by anyone. In the Americas, the knowledge of medicinal plants allowed people to thrive in great cities in the Amazon 2,500 years ago, despite not leaving a written body of knowledge.

In the previous chapter we covered the most bioactive ones available to us in the West. One important way these remedies upgrade your brain and your health is by eliminating senescent or "zombie" cells.

Senescent Cells

Senescence (from the Latin for "old") is a biological process where cells lose their ability to divide and grow. It's actually a tumor-suppressing mechanism to prevent the spread or metastasis of cells with miscoded DNA. You have more than 20,000 genes in your DNA that must be copied faithfully from mother to daughter cell, as your body is always regenerating tissues (a generation of skin cells is around seven days, and a generation of gut-lining cells around three days).

The more toxins that we are exposed to, the more "noise" in the system. Imagine someone whispering a secret to you in a crowded restaurant. The more "noise" the more that coding errors occur, and the more senescent cells are created. As we age, our bodies become less efficient at eliminating senescent cells, for these cells do not undergo apoptosis, the suicide program. They cannot be recognized by the immune system, leading to a growing population of aged cells that defy dying. Senescent cells produce chronic inflammation and contaminate their neighbors, turning them into neutered, bloated cells like themselves.

According to the World Health Organization, 100 years ago life expectancy at birth for the world population was 33 years of age, which has increased to more than 80 years today.[2] This more-than-doubling of the human life span has been accomplished through better nutrition, hygiene, and sanitation. But now that we have long lives, we are exposed to higher amounts of poisons in our food and water and air. These toxins can interfere with the accuracy of DNA copying, increasing "noise" in the cellular environment.

Researchers have found that long-lived Chinese women have reduced "noise" in crucial parts of their genome. This discovery, published in *Aging Cell*[3] connected the buildup of epigenetic "noise" to age-related conditions such as AD. By examining cell samples from various age brackets, the team observed that although entropy in the form of "noise" generally increases with age, those with the longest life span showed noise levels comparable to individuals 40 years younger. And the "noise" is caused by the toxins in the food we eat and the water we drink.

In the early 1960s, researcher Leonard Hayflick, Ph.D., along with his colleague, Paul Moorhead, Ph.D., proved that the long-held belief that human cells could replicate infinitely was wrong. Once cells have divided around 50 times, they reach what's known as the Hayflick limit and become senescent—accumulating in tissues throughout the body. If not eliminated, they reduce our ability to recover from illnesses and accelerate aging. In the brain, they cause inflammation and impair cognitive abilities. Eventually, senescent cells cause the cancers they're meant to prevent.

When we're young, our body can readily eliminate aging cells via apoptosis. This is nature's kill switch, controlled by the mitochondria in our cells. But the mitochondria in senescent cells have disabled their suicide switch. These mitochondria become big, fat, and bloated and produce a flood of free radicals that damage nearby cells—like a moldy strawberry that spoils all the others in the bowl.

Apoptosis enables your body to rid itself of as many as 10 billion aging cells every day, making room for new, healthy cells. Imagine what happens when these aging cells accumulate in your organs and tissues!

The Power of Quercetin to "Kill Zombies"

Stopping the "zombie invasion" of senescent cells becomes increasingly important as we age. Dr. James Kirkland, a geriatrician at the Mayo Clinic claimed he had gotten tired of prescribing wheelchairs and walkers to his patients and wanted to test if it was possible to slow down or reverse the aging processes that lead to decrepitude and age-related health issues. He postulated that quercetin (a flavonoid and pigment found in berries, apples, and red wine) and dasatinib (a drug used in chemotherapy to treat leukemia) could be effective at eliminating senescent cells. The story of this discovery is a reminder of the challenges researchers face in trying to study the plant medicines nature provides us.

No pharmaceutical company wanted to fund the research, because quercetin, being a natural product available everywhere, could not be patented, so there was no potential for profit. Also, pharmaceutical companies aren't enthusiastic about "once and done" interventions, which a quercetin-based treatment could turn out to be. The Mayo Clinic, being a financially independent medical center, agreed to sponsor Kirkland's research. Even so, Kirkland had bureaucratic hurdles to overcome. He was ordered by the FDA to declare quercetin a drug and demonstrate that it was safe (even though it is available in every health food store in the United States). He also had to find an inexpensive source of dasatinib, manufactured by Bristol-Myers Squibb, which was charging $367 for a one-day supply. Indian manufacturers offered to produce dasatinib for $4 per day, but Bristol-Myers Squibb refused to allow them to do so.

In 2019, Kirkland and his team were able to conduct a pilot study with patients suffering from idiopathic pulmonary fibrosis. IPF is a fatal lung condition in which the interior of the lung hardens with scar tissue. Treatment is limited; patients will need a lung transplant typically within five years. Kirkland reports: "Our study supports feasibility and provides initial evidence that senolytics may alleviate physical dysfunction in IPF."[4]

I watched my father waste away with this disease, toward the end inhaling each breath forcefully yet not able to absorb any life-giving oxygen through his scarred alveoli, the tiny air sacs in the lung that allow for releasing CO_2 and absorbing oxygen.

We have about two liters of oxygen in our body at any given time, which is why free divers are able to hold their breath for upward of 10 minutes. Out of curiosity, I tried exhaling all the breath in me and watching how long I could hold my breath with my lungs empty, with no oxygen flowing into my system. I lasted all of 20 seconds before I forcefully inhaled. And I realized that this was how my father experienced every breath.

I wish I knew back then what I know today of senolytics.

The Discovery of Senolytics, the Zombie Killers

Building on Kirkland's research, the Mayo Clinic team found that dasatinib and quercetin also eliminated senescent cells in patients with kidney disease—with only 11 days of treatment![5] The combination of these two products resulted in marked physical improvement of all the patients in the study, an extraordinary feat given the terrible prognosis that this disease carries.

The senolytic treatments that Dr. Kirkland discovered promise to delay or prevent the onset of the age-related ailments. And while senolytics also seem to increase total life span, they certainly increase the healthy years of life in laboratory animals. In effect, cardiac function in old mice given senolytics improved significantly five days after a single treatment, while mice that had a limb exposed to deadly radiation increased their exercise capacity in seven months after a single dose![6]

Eliminating senescent cells is the medicine of the future. Dr. Kirkland claims, "These agents may one day be used for treating cardiovascular disease, frailty, loss of resilience, neurodegenerative disorders, bone and joint disorders, and adverse phenotypes related to chronologic aging. Theoretically, other conditions such as diabetes and metabolic disorders, visual impairment, chronic lung disease, liver disease, renal and genitourinary dysfunction, skin disorders, and cancers could be alleviated with senolytics."[7]

Kirkland's team found that senolytics continue acting for many weeks after the medicine is no longer present, *even after administering a single dose*! There are no medications that continue to act after the drug is no longer on board. If senolytics work months or even years after a single treatment—what if you only need a treatment once a year to have its benefits be ongoing?

Senolytics appear to signal senescent cells to flip on their "suicide switch," namely apoptosis, at doses that can't be explained by a strictly chemical "killing" effect. There is no toxic poison circulating through the body and targeting old decrepit cells. You can obtain quercetin in any health food store or on the Internet. But what if you do not have access to the anticancer drug dasatinib? Well, there is a natural option that seems to be effective. It's fisetin, made from strawberries. These two naturally occurring products are known to be most effective senolytics. They are nature's remedy, available to you now! When our nomadic hunter-gatherer ancestors ate ripe berries at the end of summer, they were ingesting senolytics, which allowed them to eliminate senescent cells that had accumulated during the year, as well as treat many ills before they turned into serious disease. (I use quercetin and liposomal fisetin, which is up to 25 times more bioavailable than ordinary fisetin.)

THE LOS LOBOS SENESCENT CELL PROTOCOL

In my work as director of the Los Lobos Spa—our shamanic retreat center in the mountains in Chile—we have been experimenting to find the best and most effective senolytic formula. This is the protocol we developed and tested with participants in our one-week Grow a New Body program and they experienced the remarkable effects for themselves.

Twice a year, for five days, I take these supplements daily. The fisetin and quercetin are the senolytics. The other supplements support the liver and transport senescent cells out of the body.

Senolytics:

- 250 mg fisetin (liposomal) in the morning and 250 mg in the evening with food
- 1,000 mg quercetin in the morning and 1,000 mg in the evening with food
- Liver support in the evening with food:
    - 2,000 mg magnesium citrate
    - 50 mg zinc
    - 5,000 mcg B_{12}
    - 1,000 mg liposomal glutathione

Note: Discontinue the protocol if you experience diarrhea or gastrointestinal discomfort.

When James Kirkland, together with a group from the Scripps Institute, set out to find the most potent senolytics in nature, they discovered that at the very top was fisetin. They concluded: "Fisetin reduced senescence markers in multiple tissues, consistent with a hit-and-run senolytic mechanism. . . . Administration of fisetin to wild-type mice late in life restored tissue homeostasis, reduced age-related pathology, and extended median and maximum lifespan." The investigators went on to state, "Late life intervention was sufficient to yield a potent health benefit."[8]

"Hit-and-run" interventions—not the usual pharmaceutical "for the rest of your life" interventions—turned out to be powerfully effective, even late in life (read after the age of 35). At Los Lobos Spa we have noted benefits for our participants, from alleviating the symptoms of long COVID to helping restore immune balance. And the question you want to ask, of course, is why doesn't your doctor know about this? Well, now you know about it!

I want to share with you Kirkland's conclusions: "As anticipated for agents targeting the fundamental aging mechanisms that are 'root cause' contributors to multiple disorders, potential uses of senolytics are protean, potentially alleviating over 40 conditions in preclinical studies, opening a new route for treating age-related dysfunction and diseases."[9]

Where Will All the Zombies Go?

As I explained, senescent cells defy death by defeating apoptosis, the kill switch found in all cells. Kirkland and his team discovered how to eliminate zombie cells by reactivating their suicide program, and they assumed the body could easily attend to removing these dead cells and their waste products through the liver and GI tract. However, without the right transport molecules, toxins from our newly dead zombie cells may linger in our body and brain.

When we don't transport toxins out of the body, we retoxify. Garbage needs to go out. I tell my students that the most important workers in New York City after 10 P.M. are the garbage collectors. If you walk through New York at that time, you'll see bags of garbage piled up in the sidewalks, yet by 6 A.M., the garbage is gone, leaving the sidewalks clean again. When the garbage collectors go on strike in New York City, it is not good.

Our task is to support the body's extracellular matrix, the complex network that surrounds and supports cells and tissues. It regulates the flow of blood, lymph, and interstitial fluid—between blood vessels and cells—containing nutrients and holding waste products which need to be transported to the liver and out of the body.

A diet rich in fruits, vegetables, and whole grains, along with plenty of liquids to keep us hydrated, provides the necessary ingredients for the extracellular matrix to function. Hydration is particularly important in the early morning. Adults who stay hydrated are healthier, develop fewer chronic conditions (such as heart and lung disease), and live longer than those who may not get sufficient fluids, according to a National Institutes of Health study.[10] Also, certain minerals can play a role in supporting the extracellular matrix by helping maintain its structure and function. These include calcium, zinc, copper, and magnesium. Magnesium is of special concern because up to 50 percent of the U.S. population is magnesium deficient.

You will obtain the correct quantities of these minerals when you use the Grow a New Brain nutritional protocol. Next, we'll look at what's involved, including what foods you'll be eating regularly.

Key Takeaways:

We explored themes related to the importance of eliminating senescent cells. Here are some key points:

1. The importance of a diet rich in fruits, vegetables, plant-based proteins, and whole grains, along with proper hydration in supporting the extracellular matrix and overall health.

2. The role of certain minerals such as calcium, zinc, copper, and magnesium in maintaining the structure and function of the extracellular matrix.

3. The power of eliminating "zombie cells" and toxins lingering in the body.

Chapter 11

THE GROW
A NEW BRAIN
PROGRAM

In our pursuit of material facts, we often overlook the power of our dreams and their ability to fuel our imagination. Facts can provide a practical understanding of our world, yet they can oftentimes be overwhelming. When this happens, we tend to fall back on the M-brain and its set-in-stone-age beliefs. The dreams of our higher brain have the potential to inspire us, offering hope for a future that defies logical expectations yet does not deny the facts. By embracing our dreams of what we can accomplish and who we can become, we can nourish our spirit and craft a more fulfilling destiny beyond what the facts about our genetic or psychological inheritance alone may suggest.

Indigenous peoples recognize the distinction between facts and wisdom. Facts are information, such as understanding that water is composed of H_2O, or knowing a medical diagnosis. Facts are common sense. Wisdom is uncommon sense. It is the ability to make it rain or to heal yourself or others, moving beyond mere factual knowledge. It's magical and can inspire us to great feats. Sometimes, we believe this kind of wisdom is a placebo effect because it bypasses logic. Perhaps it is! Robert Buckman, an oncologist and professor of medicine at M.D. Anderson Cancer Center, points out that: "Placebos are extraordinary drugs. They seem to have some effect on almost every symptom known to mankind, and work in at least a third of patients and sometimes in up to 60 percent. They have no serious side effects and cannot be given in overdose. In short, they hold the prize for the most adaptable, protean, effective, safe, and cheap drugs in the world's pharmacopeia."[1]

By entertaining facts, which our M-brain loves because it gives it a sense of power and control, and cultivating wisdom, the quality of our higher brain, we can achieve a more creative and meaningful engagement with the world. We can come to understand that *"we are the placebo!"* as my friend Bruce Lipton likes to point out.

The Grow a New Brain program is designed to help you access the wisdom available to your higher brain, empowering you to break free from the addiction to the stress chemicals produced by our hectic lives and by our digital devices. As your brain begins generating the spirit molecule, DMT, it will unlock euphoric, transformative states of consciousness. (*Euphoria* comes from the ancient Greek for "healthy.") In these euphoric states, you will access the natural highs that our brain is wired for. Why else would we have receptors in the brain for the spirit molecules? What's more, your awareness will shift from self-centered preoccupations to a profound concern for the natural world. As wisdom unfolds naturally, you will discover fresh solutions for navigating through your daily life.

Once it is awakened, your higher brain will strive to master three timeless questions posed by every wisdom tradition:

"Who am I?"

"Where do I come from?"

"Where am I going?"

These questions need to be asked by each one of us to help us discover the meaning of our life journey. Perhaps they can never be answered fully, but that is not important. It's asking the questions that launches us on a quest of discovery and exploration of the extraordinary capabilities of our brain and our lives.

For many centuries we relied on religion to answer these questions. We learned we were the children of one god or another, that we came from dust and would return to dust or if well behaved to some heavenly realm. Then science came along and offered us better explanations: We came from a primordial bacterial soup billions of years ago, we are a collection of molecules and chemical processes, and we are going nowhere. Ancient spiritual traditions, including those that I was fortunate to be immersed in while in the Amazon, invite you instead to discover an answer for yourself. And your higher brain offers you the processing power to resolve these perennial riddles.

The higher brain helps you understand that you are not the product of a broken family; that you are not your title or name or caste; and that you are not working to achieve a goal of permanent happiness and security. Rather, you are on a mysterious journey of discovery. You realize how precious your life is. You break free of the psychological dramas that you have inherited from your family and culture, and you begin to craft a new destiny.

But to do this you have to bring your higher brain online—which is what you'll do with the Grow a New Brain program.

The 10-Day Grow a New Brain Program

This program draws on ancient nutritional and modern scientific discoveries and is a protocol you can repeat every season (I do it on solstices and equinoxes) to detoxify and upgrade your brain. The program requires six key actions, and I'll give you guidelines on how to properly prepare for each.

Caution: Do not do this program if you are pregnant or lactating, or if you have cancer, heart disease, or serious digestive issues.

Action 1: Shift out of SAD eating and into consuming organic foods.

That is, reject the standard American diet (which is "SAD"). Eat local and seasonal. Plant-based foods should be at the center of your meals, and you want to be sure you're eating enough of the power plants in this book that can turn off the genes for disease and switch on the genes for health. You want to activate your Nrf2 pathway, and the best way to do that is to eat broccoli sprouts that you grow yourself and sprinkle freely on your salads.

You'll want to eat fresh, organic produce and even start to grow some vegetables and fruits in containers or your yard. If the fresh, organic produce on your list isn't available, buy frozen versions. Avoid canned vegetables, which are loaded with sodium.

Action 2: Avoid or greatly reduce your consumption of red meat, dairy, eggs, and sugar.

Avoid red meat, dairy, and eggs to quiet your MTOR pathway. Eliminate sugar to downregulate your IGF-1 and enable your gut to repair and rebalance. Once the bad microbe population in your gut is reduced and the good microbes multiply, your digestion will improve, your immunity will become more robust, and you'll be able to manufacture serotonin for your serotonin-starved brain. Once thriving, your gut flora will more easily extract nutrients from your foods, so you will get plenty of protein from green plants, nuts, seeds, and the occasional serving of fish without feeling the need to consume red meat, dairy, and eggs, all potent dementia promoters.

Another reason to avoid eggs is that they contain estrogens, since they are produced in the hen's ovaries, which is a hormone gland. Chickens and cows want their calves and chicks to grow strong, and eggs and milk are full of growth hormones to promote this, in addition to the chemical hormones in their feed. But humans have no use for extraneous hormones that will grow tumors and damage the brain.

Remember, you want to switch your brain to run on the best possible fuel—good fat, which will help your body break down the fat around your midsection and eliminate the toxins stored there. Belly fat acts like an organ—it will manufacture hormones, especially estrogen.

Preparing for Actions 1 and 2: Clear your refrigerator and cupboards of processed foods, sugary treats, meat, dairy, and eggs. Set aside time for cooking so you aren't tempted to rely on takeout or visits to restaurants. You can cook ahead on weekends.

Action 3: Turn your kitchen into a laboratory.

I encourage you to grow your own broccoli sprouts to activate Nrf2, the master regulator of detoxification. You can purchase organic broccoli seeds through online vendors.

Use a mason jar that you will cover with muslin or cheesecloth fastened with a rubber band. Be sure you have washed the jar and sterilized it by boiling. Add 10 tablespoons of seeds in a ratio of about one part seeds to three parts water to the jar and let the seeds sit overnight away from direct sunlight to start the germination process.

The following morning, pour off the water, covering the mouth of the jar with cheesecloth held in place by a rubber band. Then, invert the jar, leaning it at a 45-degree angle inside a large bowl to ensure complete drainage. Place the sprouting jar in a dark environment (as seeds sprout best in the absence of light), such as an oven. Over the next three to four days, repeat the rinsing and draining once daily. In about five days, you'll see the flourishing of your sprout garden! Incorporate the sprouts in your salads and as a garnish in your soups. They will last about four or five days in the refrigerator.

Preparing for Action 3: You'll want to gather some simple equipment for growing sprouts and preparing *Saccharomyces boulardi*, the powerful probiotic yeast that will clear *Candida albicans* out of your gut. You will need a couple of mason jars, cheesecloth, and some rubber bands.

Action 4: Fast overnight every night.

Limit your eating to a six- to eight-hour window, or simply close your kitchen after dinner and avoid eating until midmorning. You'll cue your body to go into ketosis with your brain running on fat instead of sugar. You'll switch on autophagy, which frees up proteins stored in the recycling bins inside every cell in your body, reducing your need to consume additional protein in your meals.

Preparing for Action 4: You might be eating late at night because you're not getting enough nutrient-dense, satisfying foods during the day—or because you are bored and seek comfort foods. The good news is that your cravings for comfort foods are likely to diminish after you've been through the program, your taste buds have adjusted, and your gut flora has improved. Remember that you really don't want that sugary snack. It's the *Candida* in your gut that is sending messages to your brain that if you don't feed it sugar it will make you very unhappy.

I like to have dinner early, around 6 P.M., and then not eat anything until late morning—but if you can make it to noon without eating anything that has sugar or turns to sugar, all the better. I try to adhere to this schedule year-round. if I am not doing the 10-day program and I wake up famished, I will eat a half avocado in the morning. An avocado, roasted almonds, or a piece of wild-caught salmon (which contains good fats) will not shut down autophagy.

Action 5: Take a curated selection of supplements.

We take far too many supplements in America. For 10 days, you'll take a few key supplements daily, then a select number of maintenance supplements after you complete the program. You will then use the power plants and recipes in the Appendix to support your health and maintain clear mind.

Preparing for Action 5: When you review the supplements list for this program on page 170, notice that some supplements should be taken with food for better absorption and to avoid nausea. Make your supplement plan ahead of time so that during the 10 days of the program, you'll be prepared.

Action 6: Protect your brain through simple lifestyle activities: exercise, stress reduction, meditation, and intellectual challenges.

Preparing for Action 6: Set aside time in the early morning for stretching, yoga, hiking, or biking before you begin your busy day. Make your exercise a priority!

How Does the Grow a New Brain Program Work?

1. For 10 days, you are going to be eating real foods—a plant-based diet and taking supplements that repair and upgrade the brain. You will heal your body with food, the best medicine!

2. You can expect to reduce or eliminate allergies, postnasal drip, help with insomnia, and clear the brain fog. Many participants in this program improve more than 70 percent of their symptoms in the first week!

3. Follow these principles: Eat organic and for color, consuming five to six portions of vegetables daily. Keep your bowels moving!

4. Your meals will be 80 percent vegetables (good carbs loaded with fiber), including olives, algae, garlic and onions, asparagus, broccoli, and cruciferous vegetables. The other 20 percent will be good fats, including avocados, nuts, olive oil, coconut oil, MCT oil, and nut butters. Believe it or not, fats are good for you—if they are the right kinds of fats. These include extra virgin olive oil, coconut oil, and DHA, all of which help protect the brain.

5. Yes, you can have an optional small portion of wild-caught fish three times during the program, on the days of your choosing. You won't be eating any foods from land animals (no eggs, dairy, red meat, chicken, and so on).

6. Choose as many organic foods as possible, selecting seasonal vegetables for salads, soups, and stir-fries (frying with coconut oil). My *Grow a New Body Cookbook* is chock-full of recipes you can incorporate into the program.

7. You'll detoxify your kitchen and your body. To detoxify your kitchen, you will:

   - get rid of junk food and anything that has sugar or ingredients you cannot pronounce or that your grandmother would not have recognized

   - get rid of everything that has artificial coloring or preservatives

   - get rid of sports drinks, sodas, juices, and anything with sugar

To detoxify your body, you will:

- eliminate all dairy products, including yogurt and eggs

- eliminate all alcohol

- eliminate hydrogenated vegetable oils, including corn, sunflower, soy, and canola

- eliminate sugar and artificial sweeteners

- eliminate coffee for 10 days

- eliminate gluten-containing grains (wheat, barley, and rye, for example)

If you have trouble seeing how you can get through 10 days without coffee, use the following formula. Two days before the start of the program, cut your coffee intake by half. The next day, cut it in half again. Use green tea—not decaf coffee—as a substitute.

You'll want to eliminate gluten for the 10 days, because the body does not recognize the gluten protein (which creates inflammation) and because gluten-containing foods turn into sugar in your gut. A slice of white bread raises your blood sugar more than a spoonful of white sugar. And you might have a gluten sensitivity but not realize it. Symptoms include brain fog, joint pain, headache, fatigue, cravings, leaky gut, and bloating.

8. Break your fast late morning with a green juice! Lunch and dinner can include baked or steamed veggies and a portion of quinoa. Snack on nuts during the day.

9. Exercise 20 minutes per day and meditate for 10 minutes before bed. Options like brisk walking, cycling, or treadmill jogging can be great choices. Your target heart rate is 180 minus your age. Exercise increases the volume of the brain areas that are most important in memory: the hippocampus and the prefrontal cortex.

10. Drink 10 glasses of water during the day, helping you keep your bowels moving so you do not "retox." Note that magnesium citrate can keep your bowels moving.

11. Know the signs of retox, and be gentle with yourself. When you detoxify the body and brain, your elimination system can get overwhelmed. Signs of retox are headache, nausea, and brain fog. If you have any of these, take a day off the program and eat a healthy meal or a piece of fruit that will shut down autophagy. The first four or five days of the program can be hard, and you might feel very tired the first time you follow the protocol. After day 5, your brain fog will clear, and you will begin to feel amazing!

12. Dealing with Detox Discomfort: If you have been consuming a lot of sugar, alcohol, or dairy, you may experience some withdrawal symptoms. The key to managing these symptoms is to drink plenty of water during the day to flush out your system.

13. Start the program and supplements on a Friday. That way, you will be able to rest as needed on Saturday and Sunday. Remember: The first few days can be challenging but rewarding!

14. Stop the supplements on day 10 and continue to eat a primarily plant-based diet.

As you prepare for the Grow a New Brain program, keep in mind that you should *not* do it at the same time that you follow the Senescent Cell Protocol in Chapter 10. Wait at least two weeks between these two programs. If possible, begin the program on the day of the full moon to set your rhythms with nature. Your body is mostly water, which responds to the cycles of the moon.

What to Do Just Before Starting the Program

During the week before beginning the Grow a New Brain program, eat fewer foods that may contain allergens, including gluten-foods and dairy products. Assume that you are gluten sensitive, as most of us are, even if we do not have celiac disease. And assume that you're dairy sensitive too.

Eliminate sugars and discontinue the use of artificial sweeteners. Avoid pasta and breads made from highly processed flour, opting instead for products containing whole grains—"made with" whole grains might mean they started with whole grains and processed them anyway!

Start to phase in more vegetables and whole fruits. These recommendations will likely result in weight loss, and remember, excess body fat enhances inflammation and serves as a storage depot for many of the environmental toxins to which we are exposed.

Begin to incorporate healthy fats into your diet for optimal brain health. Despite common misconceptions, fats are essential for brain function. It's important to focus on the quality of fats consumed, not just the quantity. Avoiding hydrogenated and saturated fats and vegetable oils, as they negatively impact brain health, increasing the risk of conditions like cognitive impairment and coronary artery disease. Instead, prioritize good fats, such as avocados, nuts, extra virgin organic olive oil, and essential DHA supplements for brain support.

Supplements to Take During the 10-Day Grow a New Brain Program

- DHA: 2,000 mg daily. DHA is best taken in the evening, with or without food. Keep it refrigerated.

- B-vitamin complex containing B_{12}.

- Olive Oil: Extra virgin, organic, douse freely on salads and veggies.

- Alpha Lipoic Acid: 600 mg daily, 30 minutes before dinner or on an empty stomach before bed.

- MCT Oil and Coconut Oil: 1 tablespoon each morning.

- Broccoli Sprouts: 20 grams (a small bunch) each day with salad. Chew well. Four or five days on, two days off. Repeat.

- Curcumin (from turmeric extract): 250 mg capsule each morning and evening with or without food.

- Pterostilbene (pronounced tero-STILL-bean): 50 mg each morning and evening with or without food.

- Liposomal Glutathione: 1,000 mg morning and evening on an empty stomach.

- N-Acetyl Cysteine: 600 mg in the evening with food.

- Magnesium Citrate: 2,000 mg in the evening before dinner.

- Zinc: 50 mg in the evening with or without food.

- 5-HTP: 100 to 200 mg in the evening with food.

- *S. boullardi* Probiotic: 1 tablespoon morning and evening before food.

Supplements to Take after Completing the 10-Day Grow a New Brain Program

After completion of the program, you'll want to consider the following regimen of daily supplements.

- Multivitamin Supplement with B Complex: Take daily in the morning with or without food.
- Vitamin D_3: 10,000 IU. Take daily in the morning with or without food.
- DHA: 2,000 mg. Take daily; best taken in the evening with or without food. Keep refrigerated.
- Broccoli Sprouts: 20 grams (a small bunch) each day with salad. Chew well. Take for four or five days on, two days off, once per month.
- *S. boulardii* Probiotic: Take in the evening with or without food.

Perhaps one of the most important supplements we can have daily is sunshine. We think of the sun as providing vitamin D and a nice tan. But we need the sun. We spent millions of years under the sun, and the early morning and early evening light regulate all of the rhythms and biological clocks in our body. I love to practice the meditation below . . .

SUNLIGHT

People have enjoyed sunlight for therapeutic purposes for thousands of years. The Ebers Papyrus, an Egyptian medical text dating back to around 1550 B.C.E., contains references to heliotherapy for treating skin conditions and other ailments. The Greek physician Hippocrates, regarded as the father of Western medicine, recommended exposure to sunlight for healing all kinds of conditions. In Rome, solariums, open-air enclosures for sunbathing, were used for therapeutic and relaxation purposes. In Ayurvedic medicine, sunlight is considered one of the elements essential for balancing the body and promoting well-being. In the 19th and early 20th centuries, heliotherapy gained popularity and was important in the treatment of tuberculosis during the early 20th century.

Today, the benefits of sunlight have been eclipsed by the need for sun protection. We live a large percentage of our lives indoors and lather ourselves with sunblock whenever we go outside, terrified of skin cancer. Yet the rate of skin cancer among Australian Aboriginal peoples who spend their entire lives in the sun is a fraction of what it is for Westerners. Could it be because they have not been exposed to the toxins and assaults on their brains that we have?

EXERCISE: SUNBATHING

Spend at least 20 minutes in the sun daily, preferably in the early morning or late afternoon.

In the winter, use a full-spectrum light indoors.

OLIVE OIL: A SOURCE OF PHENOLICS

Did you ever wonder how olive oil can be "virgin" and even "extra virgin"?

Extra virgin olive oil contains compounds called phenolics that are extraordinary antioxidants, have antimicrobial properties, and protect you from toxic molecules. In Greece, Turkey, and other parts of the Mediterranean where olive trees have grown for thousands of years, oils were once extracted with hot water after the fruit was picked and crushed, which damaged the phenols. Today, growers extract the oil from the fruit while keeping the phenols intact by spinning the oil in centrifuges at ambient temperatures (using no chemical solvents). Oils processed this way can be called "extra virgin."

KITCHEN LABORATORY RECIPES: PROBIOTIC TO CLEAR OUT *CANDIDA*

Clearing *Candida* from your gut can be challenging once it has established itself. Examine your tongue in the mirror this evening and look for a whitish film on it, as this is a sign of *Candida* overgrowth. The most effective strategy for eliminating *Candida* is cutting out sugars, which serve as its primary food source, and introducing *Saccharomyces boulardii*, a beneficial yeast that will compete against *Candida* and displace it from your system.

Prior to taking *S. boulardii*, you should eliminate sugar from your diet to avoid experiencing bloating and cramps. If you are immunocompromised or have Crohn's disease, refrain from using this probiotic. Instead, consider a gentler approach by incorporating fermented foods into your diet while eliminating sugar, and consult with your doctor to determine the best course of action for your health.

If you're planning on taking *S. boulardii* in supplement form, be aware that the organisms within the capsules are dehydrated. When ingested, they will rehydrate in your stomach, which is acidic, causing them to rupture. I prefer to awaken them from their sleep by cultivating them in my kitchen laboratory, utilizing overripe, organic fruit. Frozen blueberries and raspberries are my favorites, but any very ripe fruit, such as pears, mangos, or frozen berries, will work well.

Use springwater when preparing your probiotic batch to prevent contamination by chlorine and other chemicals found in tap water.

Kitchen equipment you will need:

A blender

A saucepan

A large bowl

An oven (keep off)

Ingredients:

4 cups (400 g) organic, ripe fruit, pitted but not peeled

1 cup (237 ml) springwater

2 gelatin capsules *S. boulardii*

Put the fruit and springwater in a blender and blend for 30 seconds. Transfer the mixture to a saucepan and bring it to a boil. Let it simmer for 20 minutes. Once the mixture reaches body temperature, carefully pour the mixture into a large bowl, filling it halfway. Keep in mind that the batch will expand as it ferments, so provide ample room for growth. Add the contents of the gelatin capsules.

Place the bowl inside your oven, but don't turn on the oven; use only the oven light during wintertime. The heat from the oven light will maintain the mixture at body temperature for the next two to three days. Observe as your *S. boulardii* batch grows and ferments, creating potent medicine for your use.

After two to three days, the *S. boulardii* will have fermented all the sugars in the fruit. You might want to taste it on the second day. When there is no lingering sweet taste, you'll know it's ready.

Transfer the mixture to the refrigerator. Take one tablespoon daily before eating any food. Your *S. boulardii* will remain viable in the refrigerator for two weeks, thanks to the small amount of alcohol in the batch, which acts as a preservative. Additionally, after preparing a batch, you can utilize a spoonful of your *S. boulardii* as a starter for the next batch or use the gelatin capsules once again.

Key Takeaways:

We explored themes related to the Grow a New Brain program. Here are some key points:

1. How shifting away from the standard American diet to organic foods, emphasizing plant-based foods, can help activate genes for health.

2. Fast overnight every night for a six- to eight-hour window, promoting ketosis and autophagy and reducing the need for excessive protein consumption.

3. The Grow a New Brain program is a detoxification and brain upgrade program, emphasizing six key actions to detoxify and upgrade the brain.

   • Shift out of the standard American diet and into organic eating.

   • Avoid or greatly reduce consumption of red meat, dairy, eggs, and sugar.

   • Get vital nutrients from plants that activate the Nrf2 pathway by consuming broccoli sprouts, coffee, blueberries, and green tea.

   • Fast overnight, limit eating to a six- to eight-hour window, and avoid consuming sugar-containing foods.

   • Detoxify the kitchen by eliminating junk food, items with ingredients you cannot pronounce, sugary foods and drinks, and artificial coloring and preservatives. Next, detoxify the body by eliminating dairy, alcohol, hydrogenated oils, sugar, gluten, and coffee for a period of 10 days.

Chapter 12

AFTER GROW
A NEW BRAIN,
THE BEYOND

Our bodies and brains have become a toxic wasteland with forever chemicals and food preservatives that refuse to leave, even when we die. Like the French fries lost under the seat of your car that remain intact for years, no self-respecting bacteria is willing to eat them; cemeteries in the Western World are finding that upwards of 50% of the bodies buried there are not decaying. [1]

How you detoxify today will allow you to be recycled organically, returning to Mother nature that which has always belonged to her. My favorite intervention for whole body detoxification—other than what I eat—is known as *apherisis,* where toxins including heavy metals, microbes and viruses, and abnormal cells and proteins are filtered out of your blood. It is widely practiced in Germany and Switzerland, and has been in use for more than half a century, primarily for dialysis and treating autoimmune conditions. New technology makes it far less invasive, and the Europeans have discovered how to do so while keeping all of your plasma. It accomplishes in a couple of treatments what can take months to do through diet-based detoxification. And detoxifying the brain will not only help you live better, but also die gracefully.

Taking It with you

I've heard it said that on the other side of life, you are going to find whatever you believe in: heaven, or hell, or nothing at all. I can't say whether that is true, but I do know this: You can explore this territory personally after you detox and bring your higher brain online. And if you don't explore it now or in the near future, you will only have the opportunity to do so later, at the end of your life.

I asked one of the Amazon elders what was the most important teaching of their wisdom traditions, and she replied, "To learn how to get out of this life alive." Be this what it may, I would like to share with you an ancient and well-kept secret. Fasting for food and drink will allow you to live this life on your terms and eventually leave it with dignity—not struggling for one last breath. VSED, or voluntarily stopping eating and drinking, can be used when you are near the end of life. It will enable you to escape much suffering. And today many of us are caring for aging parents and loved ones that could benefit from knowing about this practice.

VSED is the ultimate fasting protocol and a strategy to avoid unwanted and sometimes painful life-prolonging measures. Its benefits are that you or your loved one is able to stay home and not have the stressor of being in a hospital surrounded by doctors and nurses. It requires no interventions by lawyers or signing medical releases. And it allows you or your loved one to have a peaceful passing, and on your or their own terms. VSED allows one to most often leave the body peacefully during sleep. One author claims that "this is a clinically validated exit option that enables a good quality death."[2]

There is much contemporary anecdotal evidence that describes VSED as being peaceful, painless, and dignified. The average time of ceasing body function after stopping eating and drinking is around seven days. When you ask one hundred hospice nurses to score the quality of a person's death on a scale from 0 (very bad death) to 9 (very good death,) the median score for VSED deaths, as rated by the nurses, is 8—an exceptional score that would never happen in a hospital setting hooked up to tubes and monitors. This was reported in an article in the prestigious *New England*

Journal of Medicine.[3] The nurses noted that patients "usually die a 'good' death within two weeks after stopping food and fluids. . . . The nurses rated the last two weeks of life as peaceful, with low levels of pain and suffering."

How does this work? We know that fasting enables the body to start burning its own fat stores and enter a state of ketosis. In ketosis, the liver converts the fat around your midsection and in-between organs into β-hydroxybutyrate (β-HB), which is jet-fuel for the higher brain. Your frontal lobes light up, and you can more easily access that sense of Oneness with all and the continuity of life beyond.

As your loved one approaches the end of life, they're able to avoid the fear-based circuits in the M-brain—the ones that kept them from forgiving their ex-partner or the person who hurt them. They can reach out to loved ones with compassion and understanding. Forgiveness for oneself and others comes more easily. And according to lore, the veils between the worlds part and you understand that death is a doorway we must all pass through in our infinite journey.

So why do more people not know about VSED? It's very expensive to die in a critical care hospital, and many of us are still convinced we need to take extraordinary measures to preserve the life of a loved one. But this is changing. We are beginning to understand that we do not want to die overmedicated and hooked up to tubes; especially when a natural, dignified transition is available. Our body manufactures its own endogenous morphine to regulate pain, and the pineal gland produces DMT to help us cross the great divide consciously.

I love the parting message left by Dr. David Eddy's mother who had chosen the VSED route: "Write about this, David. Tell others how well this worked for me. I'd like this to be my gift. Whether they are terminally ill, in intractable pain, or like me, just know that the right time has come for them, more people may want to know that this way exists."[4]

VSED is not for everyone. But it is an option worth considering.

Until then (and beyond) laugh heartily and dream your world into being newly each day.

APPENDIX

Brain-, Mind-, and Mood-Enhancing Beverages

The following recipes were developed together with Hyacinth Nadine, a nutritionist and longtime member of my team.

These beverages offer a delightful way to nourish your brain by incorporating power plants, including medicinal mushrooms and adaptogens, into your daily routine. These drinks are longevity tonics that are great for promoting brain health, energy, focus, and stress relief.

Feel free to customize them to suit your taste preferences and dietary needs.

Adaptogenic Brain-Boosting Smoothie

Serves 1

1 teaspoon lion's mane mushroom powder (promotes BDNF)

½ teaspoon *Bacopa monnieri* powder (adaptogen for memory and concentration)

½ avocado

1 cup blueberries

1 tablespoon chia seeds

1 cup almond milk

1 tablespoon coconut or MCT oil

In a blender, blend all ingredients until smooth. Pour into a glass and enjoy this nutrient-packed smoothie for enhanced brain function and cognitive support.

Ultimate Clarity Tea

Serves 1

1 cup brewed green tea

1 teaspoon turkey tail mushroom powder (immune modulator)

½ teaspoon gotu kola powder (adaptogen for mental clarity)

1 tablespoon coconut oil or MCT oil

1 teaspoon lemon juice

1 teaspoon raw honey or monk fruit sweetener

Brew green tea and let it cool slightly. In a blender, combine turkey tail mushroom powder, gotu Kola powder, brewed green tea, coconut oil, lemon juice, and raw honey or monk fruit sweetener. Blend until frothy and creamy. Pour into a cup and enjoy this adaptogenic tea for mental clarity.

Focus-Enhancing Matcha Adaptogen Latte

Serves 1

1 cup coconut milk

1 teaspoon reishi mushroom powder (calming)

½ teaspoon bacopa powder

1 teaspoon matcha powder

1 tablespoon MCT oil

1 teaspoon maple syrup or honey (optional)

In a small saucepan, heat coconut milk until warm but not boiling. Whisk in reishi mushroom powder, bacopa powder, and matcha powder until well combined. Add MCT oil and sweeten with maple syrup, honey, or monk fruit sweetener, if desired. Pour into a cup and relish this focus-enhancing adaptogenic latte.

Note: This can also be prepared in a blender after warming the milk.

Stress-Relieving Reishi Hot Chocolate

Serves 1

1 cup almond milk

1 teaspoon reishi mushroom powder (calming)

½ teaspoon ashwagandha powder (adaptogen for stress relief)

2 tablespoons raw cacao powder (promotes serotonin)

1 teaspoon raw honey, maple syrup, or coconut sugar

In a saucepan, heat almond milk until warm but not boiling. Whisk in reishi mushroom powder, ashwagandha powder, raw cacao powder, and coconut sugar until well combined. Pour into a mug and savor this stress-relieving hot chocolate before bedtime or in moments of relaxation.

Note: This can also be prepared in a blender after warming the milk.

Energizing Mushroom Coffee with Coconut Oil

Serves 1

1 cup brewed coffee

1 teaspoon cordyceps mushroom powder (endurance)

½ teaspoon *Rhodiola rosea* powder (adaptogen for energy)

1 tablespoon coconut oil or MCT oil

1 teaspoon raw honey, maple syrup, or monk fruit sweetener (optional)

Brew your favorite coffee. In a blender, combine the brewed coffee, cordyceps mushroom powder, *Rhodiola rosea* powder, and coconut oil. Add honey, maple syrup, or monk fruit sweetener, if desired. Blend until frothy and creamy.

Maca Power

Serves 1

A maca smoothie is a nutritious and energizing way to start your day or recharge in the afternoon. Here's a simple recipe that combines the health benefits of maca powder with the delicious flavors of fruit and nut milk. This smoothie is not only tasty but also packed with vitamins, minerals, and antioxidants.

½ banana, preferably ripe for natural sweetness

½ cup mixed berries (such as strawberries, blueberries, raspberries)

1 tablespoon maca powder

1 cup almond milk (or any nut milk of your choice)

1 tablespoon honey, maple syrup, or monk fruit sweetener (optional)

A handful of spinach for an extra nutrient boost

A few ice cubes (for a colder smoothie)

Gather all your ingredients. If you're using fresh berries, wash them thoroughly. If you prefer a colder smoothie, use frozen bananas or berries. Add the banana, mixed berries, maca powder, almond milk, and optional honey or monk fruit sweetener to a blender. You can include leafy greens like spinach. Blend on high until the mixture is smooth. If the smoothie is too thick, you can add more almond milk to reach the desired consistency. For a colder beverage, you can add ice cubes now and blend again briefly. Enjoy!

This maca smoothie recipe is highly adaptable. You can add superfoods like chia seeds for extra fiber, protein, and omega-3 fatty acids. Nut butter can also be added for a creamier texture. Enjoy this energizing smoothie as a powerful start to your day or an afternoon pick-me-up!

The following beverages are stellar performers from my *Grow a New Body Cookbook*.

Brain Awake

Serves 1

Neurons that fire together wire together! This brain tonic contains ingredients that wake up your brain and get those neurons firing on all cylinders. It can provide sustained energy without the caffeine spike and crash, improve mental focus, increase concentration, spark creativity.

4 ounces warm almond milk

4 ounces hot water

2 tablespoons cacao

¼ teaspoon Rhodiola rosea powder

¼ teaspoon Bacopa monnieri powder

½ teaspoon lion's mane mushroom powder

½ teaspoon reishi mushroom powder

¼ teaspoon ground cinnamon

Warm almond milk on the stove and add to the blender container. Add hot water, cacao, and all the powders to the blender and blend on high for 15 seconds. Serve in your favorite mug or cup and enjoy.

BDNF Booster

Serves 1

This tonic's ingredients boost your BDNFs, brain-derived neurotrophic factors, supporting creation of new brain cells in the hippocampus. Improve your cognitive function, memory, mood, and overall brain resilience while enjoying this tasty tonic.

1 cup almond milk, warm

2 teaspoons coconut oil

¼ teaspoon ashwagandha powder

¼ teaspoon curcumin powder

¼ teaspoon ginkgo powder

¼ teaspoon *Rhodiola rosea* powder

1 to 2 teaspoons honey (optional)

Measure the almond milk, oil, and powders in a blender. Add 1 teaspoon honey (or more to taste), then mix on high speed for 20 seconds. Serve in your favorite mug or cup and enjoy.

Matcha Energy Tonic

Serves 1

Thanks to the MCT oil and the high levels of the amino acid L-theanine in matcha (a finely ground green tea), this antioxidant and chlorophyll-rich tonic provides sustained energy while boosting attention and memory. The green Matcha Energy Tonic is a nourishing and energizing start to your day, but you can also drink it for an afternoon energy boost!

1 teaspoon organic matcha powder

¼ teaspoon moringa powder

2 tablespoons water

10 ounces almond milk

1 to 2 teaspoons honey

¼ teaspoon vanilla extract

1 teaspoon MCT oil

¼ teaspoon ground cinnamon

Using a matcha brush or a whisk, whisk the matcha and moringa powders with 2 tablespoons of water in a bowl until smooth. Transfer the whisked matcha mixture to a blender, then add the almond milk, 1 teaspoon honey (or more to taste), vanilla extract, MCT oil, and cinnamon. Blend on high speed for 20 seconds. Serve in your favorite mug or cup and enjoy.

Express Yourself

Serves 1

While reishi and lion's mane mushrooms are known as the "brain shrooms" that support brain health, cordyceps is the one that will help you go the distance when you're under pressure. Drink this when deadlines are looming, your energy is waning, and you have to put your head down and get stuff done! Express Yourself helps you focus and think clearly, and it also supports your immune system, energy, endurance, and libido.

1 cup almond milk or 2 ounces almond milk if using coffee instead of espresso

1 ounce freshly prepared espresso or 1 cup organic coffee

¼ teaspoon reishi mushroom powder

¼ teaspoon lion's mane mushroom powder

¼ teaspoon cordyceps mushroom powder

Warm or froth the almond milk, then transfer it to a blender. Add the espresso and mushroom powders and blend for about 15 seconds. Pour into your favorite mug or cup and enjoy.

Golden Milk Latte

Serves 1

This soothing and relaxing beverage is perfect before bed as it calms the mind and prepares you for dream time. The warming spices aid in digestion, and turmeric is a powerful antioxidant that reduces inflammation and promotes brain health. Ashwagandha, an adaptogenic root used in Ayurvedic medicine, is calming, relieves stress, and promotes better mood and sleep.

10 ounces almond milk

1 to 2 teaspoons honey or monk fruit sweetener

½ teaspoon vanilla extract

1½ teaspoons turmeric powder

½ teaspoon ashwagandha powder

Pinch of ground cardamom

¼ teaspoon ground cloves

¼ teaspoon ground ginger

¼ teaspoon ground cinnamon

Dash of freshly ground black pepper (or 2 or 3 whole black peppercorns, ground)

Warm or froth the almond milk, then transfer it to a blender. Add 1 teaspoon honey (or more to taste), the vanilla, and the powders and spices. Blend on high speed for about 15 seconds, then pour into your favorite mug or cup and enjoy.

ENDNOTES

Introduction

1. "Amazonian Indigenous Groups Have World's Lowest Rate of Dementia," Medscape, March 10, 2022, https://www.medscape.com/viewarticle/970091.

2. "What Is Dementia? Symptoms, Types, and Diagnosis," NIH National Institute on Aging, last reviewed December 8, 2022, https://www.nia.nih.gov/health/alzheimers-and-dementia/what-dementia-symptoms-types-and-diagnosis.

3. Morris et al., "Consumption of Fish and n-3 Fatty Acids and Risk of Incident Alzheimer Disease," *Archives of Neurology* 60, no. 7 (July 2003): 940–6, https://doi.org/ 10.1001/archneur.60.7.940.

4. Anahad O'Connor, "How the Sugar Industry Shifted Blame to Fat," *New York Times*, September 12, 2016, Eat section, https://www.nytimes.com/2016/09/13/well/eat/how-the-sugar-industry-shifted-blame-to-fat.html.

5. Monya Baker, "1,500 Scientists Lift the Lid on Reproducibility," *Nature* 533 (May 2016): 452–4, https://doi.org/10.1038/533452a.

6. John S. Garrow, "How Much of Orthodox Medicine Is Evidence Based?" *BMJ* 335 (2007): 951, https://doi.org/10.1136/bmj.39388.393970.1F.

7. "What Is Alzheimer's Disease? Women and Alzheimer's," Alzheimer's Association, https://www.alz.org/alzheimers-dementia/what-is-alzheimers/women-and-alzheimer-s.

8. Maunil K. Desai and Roberta Diaz Brinton, "Autoimmune Disease in Women: Endocrine Transition and Risk across the Lifespan," *Frontiers in Endocrinology* (Lausanne) 10 (April 2019): 265, https://doi.org/10.3389/fendo.2019.00265.

9. "How Many Pills Do Your Elderly Patients Take Each Day?" HCPLive, October 4, 2010, https://www.hcplive.com/view/how-many-pills-do-your-elderly-patients-take-each-day.

Chapter 1

1. "11 Fun Facts about Your Brain," Northwestern Medicine, October 2019, https://www.nm.org/healthbeat/healthy-tips/11-fun-facts-about-your-brain.

2. "How Much Information Do We Learn Every Day?" Wonder Newsroom, April 28, 2022, https://www.blog.askwonder.com/blog/information-data-media-consumed-in-day-average.

3. Nick Bilton, "Part of the Daily American Diet, 34 Gigabytes of Data," *New York Times*, December 9, 2009, Technology section, https://www.nytimes.com/2009/12/10/technology/10data.html.

4. Michael R. Gillings, Martin Hilbert, and Darrell J. Kemp, "Information in the Biosphere: Biological and Digital Worlds," *Trends in Ecology and Evolution* 31, no. 3 (March 2016): 180–9, https://doi.org/10.1016/j.tree.2015.12.013.

5. Kristina Lerman, "The Life and Works of Hildegard von Bingen (1089–1179)," in *Internet Medieval Sourcebook* (New York: Fordham University), last modified May 24, 1995, https://sourcebooks.fordham.edu/med/hildegarde.asp.

6. Emily Willingham, "Humans Could Live up to 150 Years, New Research Suggests," *Scientific American*, May 25, 2021, https://www.scientificamerican.com/article/humans-could-live-up-to-150-years-new-research-suggests/.

Chapter 2

1. "Unique Gut Microbiome Patterns Linked to Healthy Aging, Increased Longevity," NIH National Institute on Aging, May 13, 2021, https://www.nia.nih.gov/news/unique-gut-microbiome-patterns-linked-healthy-aging-increased-longevity.

2. Scott Emerson, "The Feeling Brain: Your Enteric Nervous System," Timeless Healing, March 7, 2022, https://timelesshealing.org/2022/03/07/the-feeling-brain-your-enteric-nervous-system-7-march-2022/.

3. Green et al., "Dietary Restriction of Isoleucine Increases Healthspan and Lifespan of Genetically Heterogeneous Mice," *Cell Metabolism* 35, no. 11 (November 7, 2023): 1976–95, https://doi.org/10.1016/j.cmet.2023.10.005.

4. "1 in 3 Adults Don't Get Enough Sleep," Centers for Disease Control and Prevention, February 18, 2016, https://archive.cdc.gov/www_cdc_gov/media/releases/2016/p0215-enough-sleep.html.

5. Danny Sullivan, "Does DNA Repair Explain the Link between Sleep and Longevity?" Longevity.Technology, updated April 7, 2022, https://www.longevity.technology/does-dna-repair-explain-the-link-between-sleep-and-longevity/.

Chapter 3

1. Jonas Salk, "Human Intelligence," in *Millennium: Glimpses into the 21st Century*, ed. Alberto Villoldo and Ken Dychtwald (Los Angeles: J. P. Tarcher, 1981), 47.

2. Salk, "Human Intelligence," 52.

3. Douglas P. Fry and Geneviève Souillac, "Peaceful Societies Are Not Utopian Fantasy. They Exist," *Bulletin of the Atomic Scientists*, March 22, 2021, https://thebulletin.org/2021/03/peaceful-societies-are-not-utopian-fantasy-they-exist/.

4. Alex Hern, "US Army Retreats from Twitch as Recruitment Drive Backfires," *Guardian*, U.S. edition, U.S. News section, July 23, 2020, https://www.theguardian.com/us-news/2020/jul/23/us-military-tactically-withdraws-from-game-streaming-site-twitch.

5. Sharon Begley, "Can Meditation Change Your Genes?" *Mindful*, February 27, 2018, https://www.mindful.org/can-meditation-change-genes/.

6. Caleb E. Finch, "Evolution of the Human Lifespan and Diseases of Aging: Roles of Infection, Inflammation, and Nutrition," Supplement, *Proceedings of the National Academy of Sciences of the United States of America* 107, no. S1 (December 4, 2009): 1718–24, https://doi.org/10.1073/pnas.0909606106.

7. Aniko Korosi and Tallie Z. Baram, "Plasticity of the Stress Response Early in Life: Mechanisms and Significance," *Developmental Psychobiology* 52, no. 7 (November 2010): 661–70, https://doi.org/10.1002/dev.20490.

8. Seymour Levine, "Developmental Determinants of Sensitivity and Resistance to Stress," *Psychoneuroendocrinology* 30, no. 10 (November 2005): 939–46, https://doi.org/10.1016/j.psyneuen.2005.03.013.

9. Eriksson et al., "Neurogenesis in the Adult Human Hippocampus," *Nature Medicine* 4 (November 1998): 1313–7, https://doi.org/10.1038/3305.

10. Michelle Z. Donahue, "Prehistoric 'Aspirin' Found in Sick Neanderthal's Teeth," *National Geographic*, March 8, 2017, https://www.nationalgeographic.com/history/article/neanderthals-teeth-diet-medicine-microbiome-humans-science.

11. Jonathan Miner and Adam Hoffhines, "The Discovery of Aspirin's Antithrombotic Effects," *Texas Heart Institute Journal* 34, no. 2 (2007): 179–86, https://www.ncbi.nlm.nih.gov/pmc/articles/PMC1894700/.

12. W. Edward Craighead and Charles B. Nemeroff, eds., *The Corsini Encyclopedia of Psychology and Behavioral Science*, 3rd ed. (New York: John Wiley and Sons, 2000), 1212.

13. Per-Henrik Zahl, Jan Maehlen, and H. Gilbert Welch, "The Natural History of Invasive Breast Cancers Detected by Screening Mammography," *Archives of Internal Medicine* 168, no. 21 (November 24, 2008): 2311–6, https://doi.org/10.1001/archinte.168.21.2311.

Chapter 4

1. Brian G. Dias and Kerry J. Ressler, "Parental Olfactory Experience Influences Behavior and Neural Structure in Subsequent Generations," *Nature Neuroscience* 17 (2014): 89–96, https://doi.org/10.1038/nn.3594.

2. Yehuda et al., "Holocaust Exposure Induced Intergenerational Effects on *FKBP5* Methylation," *Biological Psychiatry* 80, no. 5 (September 1, 2016): 372–80, https://doi.org/10.1016/j.biopsych.2015.08.005.

3. Yehuda et al., "Transgenerational Effects of Posttraumatic Stress Disorder in Babies of Mothers Exposed to the World Trade Center Attacks during Pregnancy," *Journal of Clinical Endocrinology and Metabolism* 90, no. 7 (July 2005): 4115–8, https://doi.org/10.1210/jc.2005-0550.

4. Rachel Yehuda, "How Parents' Trauma Leaves Biological Traces in Children: Adverse Experiences Can Change Future Generations through Epigenetic Pathways," *Scientific American*, July 1, 2022, https://www.scientificamerican.com/article/how-parents-rsquo-trauma-leaves-biological-traces-in-children/.

5. Dias-Ferreira et al., "Chronic Stress Causes Frontostriatal Reorganization and Affects Decision-Making," *Science* 325, no. 5940 (July 31, 2009): 621–5, https://doi.org/10.1126/science.1171203.

6. Robert Sapolsky, quoted in Natalie Angier, "Brain Is a Co-Conspirator in a Vicious Stress Loop," *New York Times,* August 17, 2009, https://www.nytimes.com/2009/08/18/science/18angier.html.

7. "Brain Scans Show Meditation Changes Minds, Increases Attention," June 25, 2007, University of Wisconsin-Madison: News, https://news.wisc.edu/brain-scans-show-meditation-changes-minds-increases-attention/.

8. Quoted by Sharon Begley in *Train Your Mind, Change Your Brain: How a New Science Reveals Our Extraordinary Potential to Transform Ourselves* (New York: Ballantine Books, 2007).

9. https://goodjudgment.com.

10. Sicher et al., "A Randomized Double-Blind Study of the Effect of Distant Healing in a Population with Advanced AIDS: Report of a Small Scale Study," *Western Journal of Medicine* 169, no. 6 (December 1998): 356–63, https://pubmed.ncbi.nlm.nih.gov/9866433/.

Chapter 5

1. Maggie Fox, "One in 6 Americans Take Antidepressants, Other Psychiatric Drugs: Study," NBC News, December 12, 2016, https://www.nbcnews.com/health/health-news/one-6-americans-take-antidepressants-other-psychiatric-drugs-n695141.

2. Tom Metcalfe, "What Made Oxford's Medieval Students So Murderous?" *National Geographic*, October 3, 2023, https://www.nationalgeographic.com/premium/article/medieval-murder-rate-students-oxford-map-coroner.

3. Joan Stephenson, "Exposure to Home Pesticides Linked to Parkinson Disease," *JAMA* 283, no. 23 (June 21, 2000): 3055–56, https://doi.org/10.1001/jama.283.23.3055.

4. Jared Diamond, "The Worst Mistake in the History of the Human Race," *Discover Magazine*, May 1, 1999, https://www.discovermagazine.com/planet-earth/the-worst-mistake-in-the-history-of-the-human-race

Chapter 6

1. Daniel P. Radin and Parth Patel, "BDNF: An Oncogene or Tumor Suppressor?" *Anticancer Research* 37, no. 8 (August 2017): 3983–90, https://doi.org/10.21873/anticanres.11783.

2. Stephen M. Rappaport, "Implications of the Exposome for Exposure Science," *Journal of Exposure Science and Environmental Epidemiology* 21 (January 2011): 5–9, https://doi.org/10.1038/jes.2010.50.

3. Hongfei Liu et al, "The effect of omega 3 supplementation on serum brain-derived neurotrophic factor: A systematic review and meta-analysis," *European Journal of Integrative Medicine*, Volume 61 (2023), 102264, https://doi.org/10.1016/j.eujim.2023.102264.

4. Yurko-Mauro et al., "O1-04-01: Results of the MIDAS Trial: Effects of Docosahexaenoic Acid on Physiological and Safety Parameters in Age-Related Cognitive Decline," *Alzheimer's and Dementia* 5, no. 4S Part 3 (July 2009): P84, https://doi.org/10.1016/j.jalz.2009.05.214.

5. Morris et al., "Consumption of Fish and n-3 Fatty Acids and Risk of Incident Alzheimer Disease," *Archives of Neurology* 60, no. 7 (July 2003): 940–6, https://doi.org/ 10.1001/archneur.60.7.940.

6. Sourav Kumar and Amal Chandra Mondal, "Neuroprotective, Neurotrophic and Anti-Oxidative Role of *Bacopa monnieri* on CUS Induced Model of Depression in Rat," *Neurochemical Research* 41, no. 11 (November 2016): 3083–94, https://doi.org/10.1007/s11064-016-2029-3.

7. Melamed et al., "The Plant Component of an Acheulian Diet at Gesher Benot Ya'aqov, Israel," *Proceedings of the National Academy of Sciences of the United States of America* 113, no. 51 (December 5, 2016): 14674–9, https://doi .org/10.1073/pnas.1607872113.

8. Weuve et al., "Physical Activity, Including Walking, and Cognitive Function in Older Women," *JAMA* 292, no. 12 (September 29, 2004): 1454–61, https:// doi.org/10.1001/jama.292.12.1454.

9. Yong Kyun Jeon and Chang Ho Ha, "The Effect of Exercise Intensity on Brain Derived Neurotrophic Factor and Memory in Adolescents," *Environmental Health and Preventive Medicine* 22, no. 27 (2017), https://doi.org/10.1186/s12199- 017-0643-6.

10. David Perlmutter and Alberto Villoldo, *Power Up Your Brain: The Neuroscience of Enlightenment* (Carlsbad, CA: Hay House, 2011), 92.

11. Andrew Newberg and Mark Robert Waldman, *How God Changes Your Brain: Breakthrough Findings from a Leading Neuroscientist* (New York: Ballantine Books, 2009), 19.

12. Newberg and Waldman, 124.

13. Morris et al., "Consumption of Fish and n-3 Fatty Acids."

14. Perlmutter and Villoldo, *Power Up Your Brain.*

Chapter 7

1. Magdeléna Vaváková, Zdeňka Ďuračková, and Jana Trebatická, "Markers of Oxidative Stress and Neuroprogression in Depression Disorder," *Oxidative Medicine and Cellular Longevity* 2015 (2015): 898393, https://doi .org/10.1155/2015/898393.

2. M. B. Yunus, "The Role of Gender in Fibromyalgia Syndrome," *Current Rheumatology Reports* 3, no. 2 (April 2001): 123–34, https:doi.org/10.1007/ s11926-001-0008-3.

Chapter 8

1. Karayol et al., "Serotonin Receptor 4 in the Hippocampus Modulates Mood and Anxiety," *Molecular Psychiatry* 26 (January 2021): 2334–49, https://doi .org/10.1038/s41380-020-00994-y.

2. Smith et al., "Molecular Imaging of Serotonin Degeneration in Mild Cognitive Impairment," *Neurobiology of Disease* 105 (September 2017): 33–41, https://doi.org/10.1016/j.nbd.2017.05.007.

3. Wong et al., "Serotonin Reduction in Post-Acute Sequelae of Viral Infection," *Cell* 186, no. 22 (October 26, 2023): 4851–67, https://doi.org/10.1016/j. cell.2023.09.013.

4. Christopher Wanjek, "Sleep Shrinks the Brain—And That's a Good Thing," *Scientific American*, February 3, 2017, https://www.scientificamerican.com/ article/sleep-shrinks-the-brain-and-thats-a-good-thing/.

5. Jenna Battillo, "The Role of Corn Fungus in Basketmaker II Diet: A Paleonutrition Perspective on Early Corn Farming Adaptations," *Journal of Archaeological Science: Reports* 21 (October 2018): 64–70, https://doi .org/10.1016/j.jasrep.2018.07.003.

6.	A. R. Mawson and K. W. Jacobs, "Corn Consumption, Tryptophan, and Cross-National Homicide Rates," *Journal of Orthomolecular Psychiatry* 7, no. 4 (1978): 227–30, https://isom.ca/wp-content/uploads/2020/01/JOM_1978_07_4_02_Corn_Consumption_Tryptophan_and_Cross-National-.pdf.

7.	"Study Finds Cancer Link for Muscle-Building Supplements," Brown University: News from Brown, April 13, 2015, https://news.brown.edu/articles/2015/04/muscles.

8.	Steven M. Weisberg, Nora S. Newcombe, and Anjan Chatterjee, "Everyday Taxi Drivers: Do Better Navigators Have Larger Hippocampi?" *Cortex* 115 (June 2019): 280–93, https://doi.org/10.1016/j.cortex.2018.12.024.

9.	Smith et al., "Homocysteine-Lowering by B Vitamins Slows the Rate of Accelerated Brain Atrophy in Mild Cognitive Impairment: A Randomized Controlled Trial," *PLoS ONE* 5, no. 9 (September 8, 2010): e12244, https://doi.org/10.1371/journal.pone.0012244.

Chapter 9

1.	"Per Capita Red Meat and Poultry Consumption Expected to Decrease Modestly in 2022," U.S. Department of Agriculture Economic and Research Service, last modified April 15, 2022, https://www.ers.usda.gov/data-products/chart-gallery/gallery/chart-detail/?chartId=103767.

2.	Górska-Warsewicz et al., "Food Products as Sources of Protein and Amino Acids—The Case of Poland *Nutrients* 10, no. 12 (December 2018): 1077, https://doi.org/10.3390/nu10121977, table 3 (Main Food Category Sources of Leucine, Isoleucine, and Valine Contribution to the Average Polish Diet), https://www.researchgate.net/figure/Main-food-category-sources-of-leucine-isoleucine-and-valine-contribution-to-the_tbl3_329647976.

3.	Kristi Wempen, R.D.N., "Assessing protein needs for performance," Mayo Clinic Health System, July 17, 2023, https://www.mayoclinichealthsystem.org/hometown-health/speaking-of-health/assessing-protein-needs-for-performance#

4.	Eli M. Swanson and Ben Dantzer, "Insulin-Like Growth Factor-1 Is Associated with Life-History Variation across Mammalia," *Proceedings of the Royal Society B: Biological Sciences* 281, no. 1782 (May 7, 2014): 20132458, https://doi.org/10.1098/rspb.2013.2458.

5.	Albena T. Dinkova-Kostova and Paul Talalay, "NAD(P)H:Quinone Acceptor Oxidoreductase 1 (NQO1), a Multifunctional Antioxidant Enzyme and Exceptionally Versatile Cytoprotector," *Archives of Biochemistry and Biophysics* 501, no. 1 (September 1, 2010): 116–23, https://doi.org/10.1016/j.abb.2010.03.019.

6.	Ye et al., "Quantitative Determination of Dithiocarbamates in Human Plasma, Serum, Erythrocytes and Urine: Pharmacokinetics of Broccoli Sprout Isothiocyanates in Humans," *Clinica Chimica Acta* 316, nos. 1–2 (February 2002): 43–53, https://doi.org/10.1016/s0009-8981(01)00727-6.

7.	Jae Kwang Kim and Sang Un Park, "Current Potential Health Benefits of Sulforaphane," *EXCLI Journal* 15 (2016): 571–77, https://doi.org/10.17179/excli2016-485.

8.	Thaler et al., "Anabolic and Antiresorptive Modulation of Bone Homeostasis by the Epigenetic Modulator Sulforaphane, a Naturally Occurring Isothiocyanate," *Journal of Biological Chemistry* 291, no. 13 (March 25, 2016): 6754–71, https://doi.org/10.1074/jbc.M115.678235.

9. Funakoshi-Tago et al., "Pyrocatechol, a Component of Coffee, Suppresses LPS-Induced Inflammatory Responses by Inhibiting NF-κB and Activating Nrf2," *Scientific Reports* 10 (2020): 2584, https://doi.org/10.1038/s41598-020-59380-x.

10. Susanna C. Larsson and Alicja Wolk, "Coffee Consumption and Risk of Liver Cancer: A Meta-Analysis," *Gastroenterology* 132, no. 5 (May 2007): 1740–5, https://doi.org/10.1053/j.gastro.2007.03.044.

11. Usharani Pingali, Raveendranadh Pilli, and Nishat Fatima, "Effect of Standardized Aqueous Extract of Withania Somnifera on Tests of Cognitive and Psychomotor Performance in Healthy Human Participants," *Pharmacognosy Research* 6, no. 1 (January–March 2014): 12–8, https://doi.org/10.4103/0974-8490.122912.

12. Hyoeun Yoo and Hyun-Sook Kim, "Cacao Powder Supplementation Attenuates Oxidative Stress, Cholinergic Impairment, and Apoptosis in D-Galactose-Induced Aging Rat Brain," *Scientific Reports* 11 (2021): 17914, https://doi.org/10.1038/s41598-021-96800-y.

13. Theophrast Paracelsus, "Die dritte Defension wegen des Schreibens der neuen Rezepte," in *Septem defensiones* (1538; Werke, vol. 2, Darmstadt: Wissenschaftliche Buchgesellschaft, 1965), 510, http://www.zeno.org/Philosophie/M/Paracelsus/Septem+Defensiones/Die+dritte+Defension+wegen+des+Schreibens+der+neuen+Rezepte.

14. Pouremamali et al., "An Update of Nrf2 Activators and Inhibitors in Cancer Prevention/Promotion," *Cell Communication and Signaling* 20 (2022): 100, https://doi.org/10.1186/s12964-022-00906-3.

Chapter 10

1. Song Xuan Ke, "The Principles of Health, Illness and Treatment—The Key Concepts from 'The Yellow Emperor's Classic of Internal Medicine,'" *Journal of Ayurveda and Integrative Medicine* 14, no. 1 (January–February 2023): 100637. https://doi.org/10.1016/j.jaim.2022.100637.

2. "Life expectancy at birth (years)," Global Heath Observatory, World Health Organization, https://www.who.int/data/gho/data/indicators/indicator-details/GHO/life-expectancy-at-birth-(years).

3. Wang et al., "Methylation Entropy Landscape of Chinese Long-Lived Individuals Reveals Lower Epigenetic Noise Related to Human Healthy Aging," *Aging Cell* 00 (April 2, 2024): e14163, https://doi.org/10.1111/acel.14163.

4. Justice et al., "Senolytics in Idiopathic Pulmonary Fibrosis: Results from a First-in-Human, Open-Label, Pilot Study," *eBioMedicine* 40 (February 2019): 554–63, https://doi.org/10.1016/j.ebiom.2018.12.052.

5. Hickson et al., "Senolytics Decrease Senescent Cells in Humans: Preliminary Report from a Clinical Trial of Dasatinib plus Quercetin in Individuals with Diabetic Kidney Disease," *eBioMedicine* 47 (September 2019): 446–56, https://doi.org/10.1016/j.ebiom.2019.08.069.

6. Zhu et al., "The Achilles' Heel of Senescent Cells: From Transcriptome to Senolytic Drugs," *Aging Cell* 14, no. 4 (August 2015): 644–58, https://doi.org/10.1111/acel.12344.

7. Zhu et al., "The Achilles' Heel of Senescent Cells."

8. Yousefzadeh et al., "Fisetin Is a Senotherapeutic That Extends Health and Lifespan," *eBioMedicine* 36 (October 2018): 18–28, https://doi.org/10.1016/j.ebiom.2018.09.015.

9. J. L. Kirkland and T. Tchkonia, "Senolytic Drugs: from Discovery to Translation," Mayo Clinic, JIM Review, https://doi.org/10.1111/joim.13141.

10. NIH National Heart, Lung, and Blood Institute, "Good Hydration Linked to Healthy Aging," *ScienceDaily*, January 2, 2023, https://www.sciencedaily.com/releases/2023/01/230102100941.htm.

Chapter 11

1. Tim Newman, "Is the Placebo Effect Real?" *Medical News Today*, September 7, 2017, https://www.medicalnewstoday.com/articles/306437#examples-of-the-placebo-effect.

Chapter 12

1. Marianne Guenot, "Dead Bodies Are Randomly Mummifying in Portugal, Baffling Scientists and Sparking a Crisis in Its Graveyards," Business Insider, November 3, 2022, https://www.businessinsider.com/unexplained-mummification-to-blame-for-portugal-graveyard-crisis-2022-11

2. Thaddeus Mason Pope and Lindsey E. Anderson, "Voluntarily Stopping Eating and Drinking: A Legal Treatment Option at the End of Life" (October 7, 2010), Widener Law Review, vol. 17, p. 363, 2011, Widener Law School Legal Studies Research Paper No. 10–35, https://ssrn.com/abstract=1689049

3. Ganzini et al, "Nurses' Experiences with Hospice Patients Who Refuse Food and Fluids to Hasten Death," *New England Journal of Medicine* 349, no. 4 (July 24, 2003), https://www.nejm.org/doi/full/10.1056/NEJMsa035086

4. David M. Eddy, "A Conversation with My Mother," *JAMA* 272, no. 3, (July 20, 1994):179–181, https://doi.org/10.1001/jama.1994.03520030013005

ACKNOWLEDGMENTS

First and foremost, I would like to extend my gratitude to my awesome editors at Hay House, Anna Cooperberg and Patricia Gift, whose keen insights have made this book possible. They knew from the start that if the brain was simple enough that we could understand it, we would be so simple that we couldn't... yet they still encouraged me in this mad endeavor that flies in the face of conventional science that until recently believed the brain could not repair or renew itself. Their attention to detail and unwavering support have been invaluable throughout this journey.

A deep bow of gratitude to my editor Nancy Peske. The book is what it is due to her tireless revision of endless versions of the manuscript and her help making the science uncomplicated.

I am grateful to my mentors and guides, who helped me navigate the stormy waters of brain science and mind-blowing ceremonies deep in the Amazon rainforest. Your wisdom and guidance have been the bedrock of my work, and I owe much of my understanding to your generous teachings.

A loving thank you to my 101-year-old mother—living proof that we can take our brains with us for our entire lives. Her indomitable spirit and intellect continue to inspire me, and her search for a man who can keep up with her zest for life never ceases to amuse and motivate me.

To my most generous friends, Mark Hyman and David Perlmutter, with whom I have co-led many retreats to heal the body and upgrade the brain. Thank you for your unwavering friendship. Your dedication to wellness and your teachings of how we can get our healthspan to equal our lifespan has enriched my life and work in countless ways.

I also extend my deepest appreciation to the sages of the Amazon and the Andes. Your guidance and knowledge of the herbs and plants that repair and regenerate the brain have been transformative. Your teachings have opened my eyes to the profound healing powers of nature, and for that I am eternally grateful.

Last but not least, to my wife, Marcela Lobos, who put up with my obsession with reading every important science paper written about the brain, and to my students who have supported me on this journey. Your encouragement and belief in my work have been a constant source of strength. Thank you for being part of this incredible journey.

ABOUT THE AUTHOR

Alberto Villoldo has trained as a psychologist and medical anthropologist, and has studied the healing practices of the Amazon and the Andean shamans. Dr. Villoldo directs the Four Winds Society, where he trains individuals in the U.S. and Europe in the practice of shamanic energy medicine. He is the founder of the Light Body School, which has campuses in New York, California, Miami, and Germany. Dr. Villoldo has written numerous best-selling books, including *Shaman, Healer, Sage*; *Grow a New Body*; *Grow a New Body Cookbook*; and *Power Up Your Brain*. Find out more at **thefourwinds.com.**

Hay House Titles of Related Interest

YOU CAN HEAL YOUR LIFE, the movie,
starring Louise Hay & Friends
(available as an online streaming video)
www.hayhouse.com/louise-movie

THE SHIFT, the movie,
starring Dr. Wayne W. Dyer
(available as an online streaming video)
www.hayhouse.com/the-shift-movie

***

GROW A NEW BODY by Alberto Villoldo

POWER UP YOUR BRAIN by Alberto Villoldo and
Dr. David Perlmutter

GROW A NEW BODY COOKBOOK by Alberto Villoldo
with Chef Conny Andersson

THE BRAIN FOG FIX by Dr. Mike Dow

MEDICAL MEDIUM BRAIN SAVER by Anthony William

All of the above are available at your local bookstore,
or may be ordered by contacting Hay House (see next page).

***

We hope you enjoyed this Hay House book. If you'd like to receive our online catalog featuring additional information on Hay House books and products, or if you'd like to find out more about the Hay Foundation, please contact:

Hay House LLC, P.O. Box 5100, Carlsbad, CA 92018-5100
(760) 431-7695 or (800) 654-5126
www.hayhouse.com® • www.hayfoundation.org

———

Published in Australia by:
Hay House Australia Publishing Pty Ltd
18/36 Ralph St., Alexandria NSW 2015
Phone: +61 (02) 9669 4299
www.hayhouse.com.au

Published in the United Kingdom by:
Hay House UK Ltd
1st Floor, Crawford Corner,
91–93 Baker Street, London W1U 6QQ
Phone: +44 (0)20 3927 7290
www.hayhouse.co.uk

Published in India by:
Hay House Publishers (India) Pvt Ltd
Muskaan Complex, Plot No. 3,
B-2, Vasant Kunj, New Delhi 110 070
Phone: +91 11 41761620
www.hayhouse.co.in

———

Let Your Soul Grow

Experience life-changing transformation—one video at a time—with guidance from the world's leading experts.

www.healyourlifeplus.com

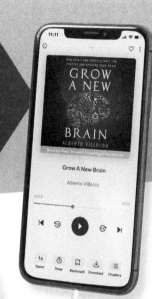
 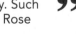

Free e-newsletters
from Hay House, the Ultimate
Resource for Inspiration

Be the first to know about Hay House's free downloads, special offers, giveaways, contests, and more!

 Get exclusive excerpts from our latest releases and videos from *Hay House Present Moments*.

 Our *Digital Products Newsletter* is the perfect way to stay up-to-date on our latest discounted eBooks, featured mobile apps, and Live Online and On Demand events.

 Learn with real benefits! *HayHouseU.com* is your source for the most innovative online courses from the world's leading personal growth experts. Be the first to know about new online courses and to receive exclusive discounts.

 Enjoy uplifting personal stories, how-to articles, and healing advice, along with videos and empowering quotes, within *Heal Your Life*.

Sign Up Now!

Get inspired, educate yourself, get a complimentary gift, and share the wisdom!

Visit www.hayhouse.com/newsletters to sign up today!